SAP BAAT LO HAN KYUN

The palms of the eighteen Lo Han

Luis Lázaro Leo

Copyright © 2018 Luis Lázaro Leo
Published by Luis Lázaro Leo

All rights reserved. It is forbidden any full or half copy of this work without the express permission of the author.

The author declines all responsibility for any injury or accident that may happen to the reader for the reading and practice of the content in this play. It is recommended to call a doctor and/or expert on the subject before any attempt of any physical activity.

SAP BAAT LO HAN KYUN The palms of the eighteen Lo Han / Luis Lázaro Leo - 1st Edition

Dedicated to my son Nil 尼你 my biggest treasure.

Thanks to Chen Huan 陈欢 "Juana" for her big effort in the help that she has offered me for the translation of the manuscript that was handed to me by my master Sifu Pun after learning the form, the manuscript that the GM Chan Yiu Chi handed to my Sigung Pun Fan father of my Sifu.

Also, to thank Sifu Rolando Martins for the photoshoot, with any doubts excellent photos to fairly Illustrate the sequence of the form.

Also, to thank Lee Wingsze 李泳恩 for her last touches in the translations.

This book has been translated by Sabahaven.

And finally I would like to thank Sifu Pun for all his teachings.

Thanks to all these collaborations this project has become a reality.

INDEX

PROLOGUE 7

1. The origin of The palms of the 18 Lo Han 8
   History of Chan Heung and the eighteen disciples 9

2. The eighteen Lo Han 10

3. The Yam Yeung theory 14
   The energy meridians 15
   The three elixir fields 16
   The three heater 18
   The three doors 20
   The 9 dragons pearls 20
   The three treasures 21

4. The Lo Han Kung system 22
   Important points for the practice of the form 22
   Sap Baat Lo Han Kyun characteristics 23
   Objective of the practice 23
   Contraindications 23

5. SAP BAAT LO HAN KYUN 24
   零. Bei Sik - Preparing 25
   一. This first palm - Chiu Tin Daap Dei - To the sky pushing the earth 26
   二. The second palm - Paao Saan Dou Hoi - To remove the mountain and to overturn the sea 28
   三. The third palm - Haak Fu Teui Saan - The black tiger pushes the mountain 32
   四. The fourth palm - Daai Paang Jin Chi - The sacred great bird opens his wings 36
   五. The fifth palm - Tung Ji Baai Gun Yam - The kid praises the Gun Yam goddess 38
   六. The sixth palm - Seung Ha Laau Jaau - Fishing in the bottom with the claws 42
   七. The seventh palm - Yap Jaau Au Jung - Greeting with the claw in the chest 44
   八. The eighth palm - Waan Gung Hoi Gaak - To tense the arc opening the diaphragm 46
   九. The ninth palm - Gam Paau Lou Jaau - The golden leopard shows his claws 48
   十. The tenth palm - Teui Lik Dong Dit - To kick with the balancing energy 54
   十一. The eleventh palm - Yi Saan Dou Hoi - To move the mountain and to overturn the sea 58
   十二. The twelfth palm - Jo Jeun Lung Taam Hoi - The great dragon searches in the sea 62
   十三. The thirteenth palm - Yau Jeun Lung Taam Hoi - The great dragons searches in the sea 66
   十四. The fourteenth palm - Jo Au Jaau Hoi - Fishing with the claw in the sea 70
   十五. The fifteenth palm - Lo Hon Saai Tou - Lo Han shows his abdomen to the sun 72
   十六. The sixteenth palm - Yau Au Jaau Hoi - Fishing with the claw in the sea 74
   十七. The seventeenth palm - Seung Jin Ji - Double arrow fingers 76
   十八. The eighteenth palm - Seung Ha Chung Kyun - Throw both fists down 78

INDEX

6. SAP BAAT LO HAN KYUN - SEQUENCE 83

7. LINEAGE 94

AUTHOR'S NOTE 96
ABOUT THE AUTHOR 97

TECHNICAL GLOSSARY 98

PROLOGUE

The Lohan Kung is one of the biggest treasures that the Choy Lee Fut system offers us. Heir of the purest Shaolin tradition, he got enriched with different influences through the succeeding generations until becoming one of the most complete Chi Kung (Qi Gong) systems that exists.

In his large work is noticeable the form of the "The palms of the 18 Lohan". Considered the seed from which the Shaolin's Kung Fu developed, it contains the essence of the whole system.

Right up to the present days it has arrived many versions of the form, transmitted by different masters and branches of the style. But now we have the privilege of knowing the original version in the exact same version that Chan Heung wrote, founder of the Choy Lee Fut.

I know Sifu Luis Lázaro from a very long time ago. I share with him the passion for martial arts and the interest for learning them and to transmit them as how they were originally created.

His continued commitment in achieving it has taking him to travel in several occasions to China in order to contact with the highest level masters in the disciplines that he practices. As an outcome of it he has managed to obtain the original manuscripts of the Choy Lee Fut system, from which the father of his master received by the hand of the GM Chan Yiu Chi, of whom he was a disciple.

It is a complete privilege that he is willing to share with us through his courses, his classes and now with his books. We have the occasion of this mythical form in the same way as it was conceived by his creator, with any tampering or interpretations. It is a luxury that we can access thanks to the effort and tenacity of Sifu Luis.

With any doubt, it is a great work that any Qi Gong, Choy Lee Fut or Wu Shu lover shouldn't miss.

Jose Beneyto

THE ORIGIN OF THE PALMS OF THE 18 LOHAN

For 9 years that the monk Bodhidarma 菩提达摩 (Daat Mo 达摩 da mo in Mandarin), dedicated to meditate in the cave, for the lack of movement and the harshness of the time he suffered fatigue, muscular pain and diseases.

During this period he was studying the animals and with his knowledge of the hindian Yoga and exercises that he learned in China based on the animals movements he codified the Chi Kung form 气功 (qi gong in Mandarin) called The palms of the 18 Lo Han (sap baat lo hon kyun 十八罗汉拳).

The Lo Han Kung 罗汉功 is the Chi Kung system created by Da Mo over 1500 years ago. This system works over the three elixir fields SAAM DAAN TIN 三丹田, the three doors of the backbone SAAM GWAAN 三关, the triple heater SAAM JIU 三焦 and the energy meridians GING LOK 经络.

During the Song 宋朝 (960-1278 A.D.) dinasty, the famous Gok Yun 觉远 monk extended the 18 excercises to 72 movements and then the Choi Gwok Yu 蔡国如, Lei Sau 李绶 and Baak Yuk Fung 白玉峯 monks extended them to 173, this movements were the basics of the Kung Fu 功夫 system, Siu Lam Kyun Faat 少林拳法 (in mandarin shao lin chuan fa), and it's said that it was the origin of the Chinese martial arts.

This Chi Kung system was kept in secret inside of the monastery until its looting and destruction.

The Choi Fuk 蔡福禅师 monk, (usually can be found written as Choy Fook) who is one of the survivors of the fire, he ran away to the Guang Dong 广东 province in the Lo Fau Saan 罗浮山 mountain. From there he travelled to Chan Heung 陈享 to become his disciple, with him he learned the Shaolin Siu Lam Kyun Faat 少林拳法 martial system, the therapeutic Chi Kung 气功 system, just like Dit Da Yun Fong 跌打丸方 and the chinese medicine.

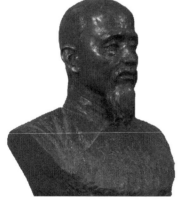

All this knowledge were collected by Chan Heung and kept saved inside of his Kung Fu Choy Lee Fut 蔡李佛 system, of which It has stayed until our present days thanks to the generations of masters that have worked to keep alive his legacy.

HISTORY OF CHAN HEUNG AND THE EIGHTEEN DISCIPLES

Chan Heung had four masters, although the most acquaintances are the first three

1. Choi Fuk 蔡福 传授
2. Lei Yau Saan 李友山 传授
3. Chan Yun Wu 陈远护 传授
4. Bak Yuk Fung Daai Si 白玉峰大师 传授

After inaugurating and structuring all his knowledge obtained in his Choy Lee Fut system, Chaan Heung obtained 18 original disciples, known as The eighteen Lohan (十八罗汉), they were the decision makers of the Choy Lee Fut system diffusion for all over the south of China.

1. Lung Ji Choi 龙子才, whom he opened a school in the Xun Zhou's city 浔州
2. Chan Din Wun 陈典桓 started the Hung Sing school in Fo Shan 佛山
3. Chan Din Yau 陈典犹 in Nan Hai 南海
4. Chan Daai Yap 陈大撑 in Guang Zhou 广州
5. Chan Din Sing 陈典成 in Zhong Shan 中山
6. Chan Mau Jong 陈谋庄 in Pan Yu 番禺
7. Chan Din Bong 陈典邦 in Dong Guan 东莞
8. Chan Din Wai 陈典惠 in Kai Ping 开平
9. Chan Din Jan 陈典珍 in Tai Shan 台山
10. Chan Syun Dung 陈孙栋 in En Ping 恩平
11. Chan Sing Hin 陈承显 in He Shan 鹤山
12. Chan Daai Ching 陈大成 in Zhao Qing 肇庆
13. Chan Sing Fong 陈承晃 in Hui Cheng 会城
14. Chan Yin Yu 陈燕贻 in Jiang Men 江门

And the next four disciples instructed in the 26 alleys in the San Wui 新会 (xin hui in mandarin)

15. Chan Daai Sing 陈大成
16. Chan Sing Din 陈胜典
17. Chan Mau Wing 陈谋荣
18. Chan Din Gung 陈典拱

THE EIGHTEEN LO HAN (Arhats): according to the Mahayana Buddhism tradition, they are the original Buda's followers and that have followed the eightfold path and reached the four stages of the illumination. They have reached the Nirvana state and they are free of earthly desires. They are in charge of protecting the Buddhist faith and to wait on earth for the arrive of Maitreya.

The legend says that the 18 Lo Han knew in 891 A.D about the calligraphy and paint skills from the Gun Yau 貫休 monk (in mandarin Guanxiu), and they appeared to the monk in a dream to ask him paint their portraits .

Due his ability to protect himself from the bad spirits, the Lo Han became in the protectors of the Buddhist temples and the main hall of every temple.

In the Chinese Tradition, the 18 Luohans are generally presented in the order they are said to have appeared to Guan Xiu, not according to their power.

The sitting on a deer Lo Han, KEI LUK LO HAN 騎鹿 罗汉

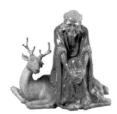

Sitting dignified on a deer,
As if in deep thought.
With perfect composure,
Contented with being above worldly pursuits.

The happy Lo Han, HEI HING LO HAN 喜庆 罗汉

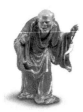

Decimating the demons,
The universe now cleared.
Hands raised for jubilation,
Be wild with joy.

The Raised Bowl Lo Han, GEUI BUT LO HAN 举钵 罗汉

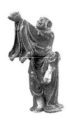

In majestic grandeur,
Joy descends from heaven.
Raised the bowl to receive happiness,
Glowing with jubilance and exultation.

The Raised Pagoda Lo Han, TOK TAAP LO HAN 托塔罗汉

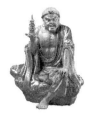

A seven-storey pagoda,
Miraculous power of the Buddha.
Forceful without being angry,
With preeminent Buddhist might.

The meditating Lo Han, JING JO LO HAN 静座 罗汉

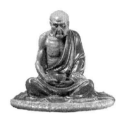

Quietly cultivating the mind,
A countenance calm and composed.
Serene and dignified,
To enter the Western Paradise.

The Oversea Lo Han, GWO GONG LO HAN 过江 罗汉

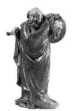

Bearing the sutras,
Sail east to spread the world.
Climbing mountains and fording streams,
For the deliverance of the humanity.

The Elephant Riding Lo Han, KEI JEUNG LO HAN 骑象 罗汉

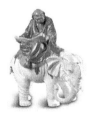

Riding an elephant with a dignified air,
Chanting aloud the sutras.
With a heart for the humanity,
Eyes scanning the four corners of the universe.

The Laughing Lion Lo Han, SIU SI LO HAN 笑狮 罗汉

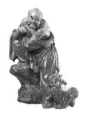

Playful and free of inhibitions,
The lion cub leaps with joy.
Easily alternating tension with relaxation,
Rejoicing with all living things.

The Open Heart Lo Han, HOI SAM LO HAN 开心罗汉

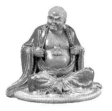

Open the heart and there is Buddha,
Each displaying his prowess.
The two should not compete,
For Buddha's power is boundless.

The Raised Hand Lo Han TAAM SAU LO HAN 探手罗汉

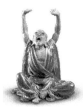

Easy and comfortable,
Yawning and stretching.
In a state of omniscience,
Contented with his own lot.

The Thinking Lo Han, CHAM SOI LO HAN 沉思罗汉

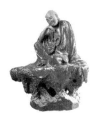

Pondering and meditating,
Understanding it all.
Above this world and free from conventions,
Compassion conveyed up to the Ninth Heaven.

The Scratched Ear Lo Han, WAAT JI LO HAN 抱耳罗汉

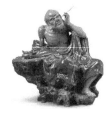

Leisurely and contented,
Happy and knowledgeable.
Full of wit and humour,
Exuberant with interest.

The Calico Bag Lo Han, BOU DOI LO HAN 布袋罗汉

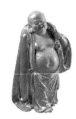

Buddha of infinite life,
Valuable bag containing secrets of heaven and earth.
Happy and contented,
Cheerful and joyful is he.

The Plantain Lo Han, BA JIU LO HAN 芭蕉 罗汉

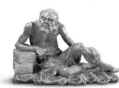

Buddha of infinite life,
Valuable bag containing secrets of heaven and earth.
Happy and contented,
Cheerful and joyful is he.

The Long Eyebrow Lo Han, JEUNG MEI LO HAN 长眉 罗汉

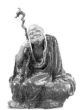

Compassionate elder,
A monk who has attained enlightenment.
Perceptive of the infinite universe,
With tacit understanding.

The Doorman Lo Han, HON MUN LO HAN 看门 罗汉

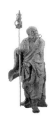

Powerful, husky and tough,
Watching with careful alertness.
With the Buddhist staff in hand.
Valiantly annihilates the evil.

The Taming Dragon Lo Han, HONG LUNG LO HAN 降龙 罗汉

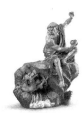

In the hands are the spiritual pearl and the holy bowl,
Endowed with power that knows no bounds.
Full of valour, vigour and awe-inspiring dignity,
To succeed in vanquishing the ferocious dragon.

The Taming Tiger Lo Han, FUK FU LO HAN 伏虎 罗汉

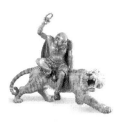

Precious ring with magical powers,
Infinitely resourceful.
Vigorous and powerful,
Subduing a ferocious tiger.

THE YAM YEUNG THEORY

The theory of Yam Yeung 阴阳 (Yin Yang in Mandarin) was the fruit of the observation of nature. The dual feature of the universe in the Chinese philosophy is assigned the concepts of Yam and Yeung. It is studied the evolution of everything as the result of the interaction of two forces, tendencies, directions, energies that are opposite to each other. The sky and the Earth, the sun and the Moon, the night and the day, man and woman, down and up, in and out, stillness and movement are just some manifestations of this intrinsic duality.

These forces cannot exist without the other, the cold cannot be defined without the heat, nor the day without the night.

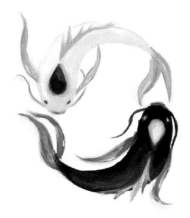

One thing, phenomenon, event, situation or object will never be total and exclusively yang or yin. For example, the day is considered yang when comparing it with the night, but the first hours of the day are yang in comparison and the hours of descent of the sun in the afternoon being still part of the day, are yin, well, the morning is yang and in the afternoon , yin inside yang.

The yin and yang are not static in time and space. The yin is transformed into yang and the yang in return evolves towards yin; The yang day will transform into the cold night yin. The evolution of the universe depends on the continual transformations of yin to yang and vice versa.

> The Dao gives birth to one.
> One gives birth to Two,
> Two gives birth to Three.
> Three gives birth to thousands of things.
> All things carry yin and embrace yang.
> When yang and yin combine, all things achieve harmony.
> *(Dao De Jing – chapter 42)*

The wise chinese observed that the inmutable in the universe is the movement. Everything moves, it transforms and changes in a permanent cycle of starts and endings where the only thing that remains is the movement. This movement has two tendencies: an expensive one or centrifuge that starts it and the other is contractive or centripetal that comes back to the origin.

THE ENERGY MERIDIANS - GING LOK 经络

Duk Mak 督脉 (Du Mai in mandarin) also called as Governor glass is the meridian located in the bottom part of the body, starts from the anus and it ends in the mouth, it has 28 points and is the channel that rule the Yang energy and the Yang meridians.

Yam Mak 任脉 (Ren Mai in mandarin) also called Conception glass is the meridian located in the frontal part of the body, it goes from the anus to the mouth, it has 24 points and it is the channel that rules the Yin energy to the Yin meridians.

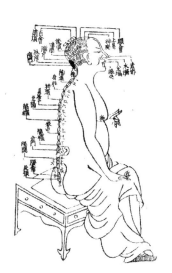
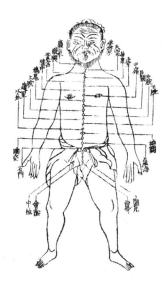

Ging Meridians 经 (Jing in mandarin)

- 12 main meridians that connect the Jong 脏 organs (liver, heart, spleen, lung, kidney and master heart) and Fu 腑 bowls (gallbladder, small intestine, stomach, large intestine, bladder, and triple heater)
- 12 different meridians that complete de main meridians, branching and reaching the places where the main meridians don't reach.
- 8 extraordinary meridians that go across with the previous meridians and help to harmonize its emptiness.

Lok Associated vessels 络 (Luo in mandarin)

12 transversal Luo that connect with the organs and gallbladder with Biao-Li relation.
- 15 longitudinal Luo that develop from the main meridians and circulate in a more superficial level.
Capillaries that come out of the Luo vessels; They are thin and small.

THE THREE ELIXIR FIELDS - SAAM DAAN TIN 三丹田

Daan Tin 丹田 (dan tian in mandarin) also translated as Cinnabar field, the old Taoist alchemist used the concept of transforming the cinnabar into gold as a metaphor of the internal energy transformation.

The Dan 丹 ideogram is the cinnabar, a mineral composed by mercury sulfide of red vermilion color that reminds the color of earth around the Yellow River which the most important symbol of the Chinese culture. And Tian 田 means agricultural fields, named to refer those energy centers where the Qi 氣 was worked at. The three Dan Tian symbolize the Sky, The Man and the Earth, those are not specific points, these are spherical area located In three parts of the body.

Low elixir field (Ha Daan Tin 下丹田) – Earth Level

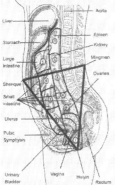

We locate two fingers under the belly button, in an acupuncture point called Qi Hai 气海 (Ren6 or Qi Ocean).

It is associated to the earth and that's the reason of the absorption and elimination of aliments, just like everything related to our sexuality.

It is the Yuan Qi 元气 (original Qi) residency place, and the first Jing 精 treasure (the essence).

Through the practice in the Chi Kung the objective is to activate it and make it stronger, as a gravity center.

Medium elixir field (Jung Daan Tin 中丹田) – Human Level

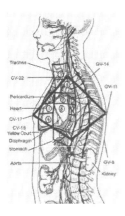

We locate it in the center of the thorax, in the level of the nipples. It matches with the Shan Zhong 膻中 point (Ren17 or Chest center)

It is associated to the man and the center that it produces and stores what proceeds of the breathed air and the ingested aliments.

Here is where the Hou Tian Qi 後天气 (acquired Qi) is stored and the second Qi 气 treasure (la energía).

Top elixir field (Seung Daan Tin 上丹田) – Sky Level

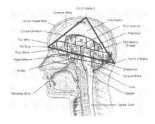

We locate the elixir field in the head, at the level of the middle of the eyebrows in the extraordinary Yin Tang 印堂 point (real seal)

The sky is associated to the brain and the senses.

This is controled by Yi 意 (Rational thought) and the third Shen 神 treasure (the spirit).

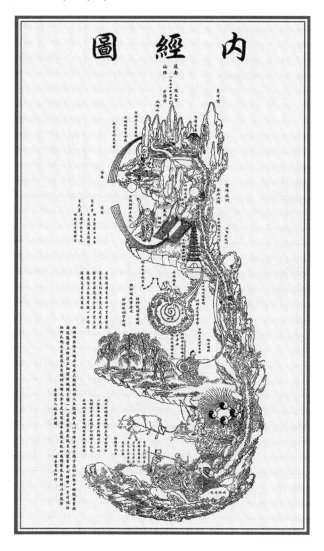

THE TRIPLE HEATER - SAAM JIU 三焦

Saam Jiu 三焦, the Chinese medicine as a multi-organ that depends on each other by an association system and it cannot be divided in individual organs as envisaged in the Western Medicine.

Its ideogram is formed by two characters: Sam 三 (San in mandarin) that means three and the chracter Jiu 焦 (Jiao in mandarin) that means heating or burning, in this way this represents the place where it's transformed o cooked through the fire. Saam Jiu is translated as Triple heater, Triple Energizer or Triple Function. The World Health Organization W.H.O decided to standardize the term Triple Energizer.

The Saam Jiu in the history of chinese medicine

In the Huang Di Nei Jing 黄帝内经 (Internal Canon of the Yellow Emperor dated around the 2600 B.C) it describes the Saam Jiu without form, but it is assigned with a meridian. It's said that its main functions are the ways of passing and the processing of liquids and food, and the organs that belong to its anatomical location are quoted.

In the Ling Shu Jing 灵枢经 (one of the two parts that establish the Huang Di Nei Jing) It is related to the metabolism of water. Is described the converging trajectories and divergent trajectories: Seung Jiu 上焦 (high heater), Jung Jiu 中焦 (medium heater) and Ha Jiu 下焦 (low heater).

The Sheng Ji Zong Lu 圣济总录 Song dinasty (960-1279) it also refers to the Saam Jiu like the channel for the liquid and food, and the place where the Qi transformations take place.

In the Nan Jing 难经 (Classic of difficulties) appear several references over the functions of the Triple heater concerning the movement and the control of all kinds of Qi, guaranteeing that this could pass through all the Fu 腑 guts and Zang 脏 organs. In the chapter 38 it is mentioned its function as governor of the Qi of the body. In the chapter 66 it is commented about its connection with the Yuan Qi 元气, transporting it from the kidneys to the internal organs. In the chapter 31 It Is confirmed its influence over the control of the Qi 元气 movement in general in all parts of the body.

The **Sueng Jiu** 上焦 is formed by the head and chest, and it includes the heart and lungs. It is characterized for his internal and rising function. From the point of view of the liquid, it is said that is like a fog. It is related to the Shen spirit.

The **Jung Jiu** 中焦 includes the solar plexus to the belly button, including the liver, stomach and spleen. It envolves the digestion, absorption and distribution functions and is related to the Qi energy.

The **Ha Jiu** 下焦 comprises the lower abdomen, including the kidneys, bladder and intestines. Function of disposal of waste, liquids and solids. It's related to the Jing essence.

The interactions between the Jing 精, the Qi 氣 and the Shen 神 are related with the internal alchemy in which the essence sublimates and rises to nourish the spirit, which generates energy. The interconnection of the Jing, Qi and Shen explains the Interconnection mind-body.

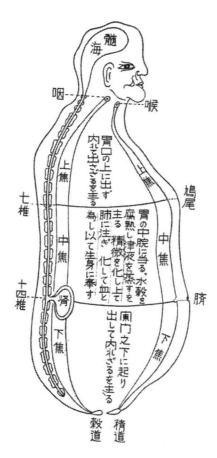

THE THREE DOORS - SAAM GWAAN 三关

Saam Gwaan 三关, according to the chinese medicine with three areas of the backbone where the energy has its entrance to the Saam Daan Tin, three elixir fields.

In the Chi Kung, to understand the concept of the three doors help to unlock the back and to raise the consciousness of the backbone, raising the Qi bloodstream.

The **Sueng Gwaan** 上关, the tall door is located at the level of the first cervical vertebra, it regulates the movement and the bloodstream of Qi 气 and Hyut 血 (Xue in mandarin, blood) from and to the head. It is related to the Shen spirit.

The associated acupuncture spot is Fung Fu 风府 (Du16 or Wind Palace), it expulses the wind to the outside and it extinguishes the inside, it nourishes the sea of the bone meadow and the brain and it opens the wholes of the Shen, the mind.

The **Jung Gwaan** 中关, the half door is located between the second and third dorsal vertebra, It regulates the movement, Qi 气 and Hyut 血 bloodstream in the area of the back, helping movement from and to the arms. It is related with the Qi energy.

The acupuncture spot associated is San Chyu 身柱 (Du12 or Pillar of the body), it relieves the heat of the Lung, it tones and eliminates the wind of the inside, it opens the wholes of the mind and It relieves the Shen.

The **Ha Gwaan** 下关, the half door is located between the third and second lumbar vertebra, it regulates the movement and the Qi 气 and the Hyut 血 bloodstream in the pelvis area, helping the movement from and to the legs. It is related with the Jing essence.

The acupuncture spot associated is Ming Mun 命门 (Du4 or Door of Life), it extinguishes the wind from the inside, it tones the Yuan Qi 元气, it removes the cold and strengthens the Duk Mak meridian, it beneficiates the Jing 精 (the essence), it clears the Shen.

THE 9 DRAGON PEARLS - LUNG DIK GAU FO JAN JYU 龙的九颗珍珠

The interconnection between the cervical area with the wrists and ankles, the dorsal area with the elbows and knees and the lumbar area with shoulders and hips is what we know as the 9 pearls. These points are reflections on each other and should be mobilized in the practice of Chi Kung as Pearls United in a rosary, so that the Union of the lumbar, dorsal and cervical with their respective reflections on the limbs have to create a harmonic movement.

THE THREE TREASURES - SAAM BOU 三宝

The Saam Bou 三宝 (in mandarin San Bao) are different states of the Qi 气 condensation:

- The Shen 神 (Spirit)
- The Qi 气 (Energy)
- The Jing 精 (Essence)

The Jing is the most dense energy, it is what we can see and touch, the Qi is the energy that moves us, the one that provides us strength and the Shen is the most ethereal and soft energy.

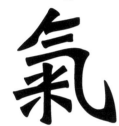

The traditional Qi character is composed by two simple characters, in one side we have the Steam 气 and for the other we have Rice 米.

The Qi can be so immaterial like the steam and at the same time so solid and dense like the rice.

The three treasures are unseparable and they need eachother to survive, the Shen promotes the Qi, the Qi charges the Jing everyday and the Jing anchors and nourishes the Shen.

From the Chinese Medicine is wanted the balance of the Three Treasures in order to assure the physical and mental well-being.

The Jing 精 (Essence), it includes all the fundamental substances of our bodies, blood, sweat, saliva, sperm, and all the group of organic liquids; it is also related with the Jing of the kidney that comes from the theory of the Earlier Heaven and the Later heaven.

The Earlier Heaven 先天元气 is the ancestral energy, our genetic material. *The Later Heaven* 后天元气 comes from the food and the air, and it recharges the Earlier Jing.

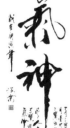

The Qi 气 (Energy),), the Qi es everything and everything is Qi, all the manifestations of nature are expressions of energy. A chinese proverb says: When the Qi clumps together, the physical body is formed; but when the Qi disperses the body dies.

The Shen 神 (Spirit) is the spiritual and emotional health, it directly influences in our physical health.

THE LO HAN KUNG SYSTEM

The Lo Han Kung system 罗汉功 works in three forms and each one of them is mainly focused in the principal work in one of the three treasures, even if the three of them simultaneously work in the three treasures because these are interconnected.

- Sap Baat Lo Han Kyun 十八罗汉拳: Work of the Jing 精 (Essence)
- Siu Lo Han 小罗汉: trabajo del Qi 气 (Energy)
- Taai Lo Han 太罗汉: trabajo del Shen 神 (Spirit)

The Sap Baat Lo Han Kyun principal work is the cultivation of the Jing, this is the reason why the principal work in this particular form is based on the stretchings. Following the Yan Yeung theory 阴阳 (Yin Tang in mandarin) this form is Yeung 阳 character, highlighting that the work in this form moves the Qi to the outside or exterior, to the muscles, tendons and joints and activates the Wai Chi 卫气 (Wei Qi in mandarin) the deffensive energy that circulates over the surface of the body.

Siu Lo Han is focused in the work of the second treasure, in this way it is worked with sequencing of continual movements and fluids where the breathing guides the movement and the movement guides the intention and concentration. This form is Yam Yeung 阴阳 character, this form moves the Qi of the Jong Fu 脏腑 (Zang fu in mandarin), the Jung (Heart, Liver, Spleen, Lung and Kidney) are the organs of Yam (Yin) character, the Fu (Small intestine, Gallbladder, Stomach, Large intestine and Bladder) are the bowels of Yeung (Yang) character.

Taai Lo Han works over the Shen, it is a form that is divided in a series of exercises that can be executed while sitting and another series can be executed while laying down, in this occasion the intention and concentration guide the breathing and the breathing guides the movement. This form is Yam 阴 character and it works over the Shen (concentration, nervous system).

IMPORTANT POINTS FOR THE PRACTICE OF THE FORM

While performing the form, the rhythm of the sequence will be always guided by the movement (jing), followed by the breathing (Qi) and for last, the intention and concentration (Shen).

The breathing must follow the movement, always inspiring through the phases of stretching and exhaling in the relaxing phases of the stretching.

It is from vital importance that in every one of the sequences has a different intention in the gazing intention phase. According the traditional Chinese medicine *The Shen can be expressed through our eyes.*

SAP BAAT LO HAN KYUN CHARACTERISTICS

This form can be performed with certain rhythm, it's not a slow execution, is a Yeung 陽 form, while performing these stretchings we have to make them in rhythm that we feel comfortable and where the breathing follow a natural rythym, we are not in a meditative form, even though the inspiring must have a slow rythym to focus in the stretching so that we can take it to its maximum elongation.

With the paractice of this form we must break into sweat while finishing it, this will indicate that the Qi has moved and that our energy has been manifested through the Yeung 陽.

OBJECTIVE OF THE PRACTICE

- Stretch the entire body, to gain flexibility, increase muscle strength and balance muscle groups.
- Prepare the tendons and muscles to prevent injury.
- Strengthen the muscular chains that protect the spine and gain flexibility to im prove its movements.
- Improve the back, stomach and kidney.
- Improve lung capacity by breathing work
- Improve the Yuan Qi 元气.
- Unlock the meridians by stretching and improving the circulation of Qi and its quality.
- Regulate internal organs and keep them healthy.
- Work the concentration and calm the mind.

CONTRAINDICATIONS

- Elderly people or with a weak physical state should practice the form smoothly and without making great efforts, the part of the balances should be done with the foot of the kick on the ground to generate stability.
- Do not practice during pregnancy.
- Do not practice when you have any type of inflammatory disease or caused by pathogenic factors.
- Do not practice in cold, windy or humid environments.

CHAPTER 5

十八罗汉拳

BEI SIK
PREPARADO

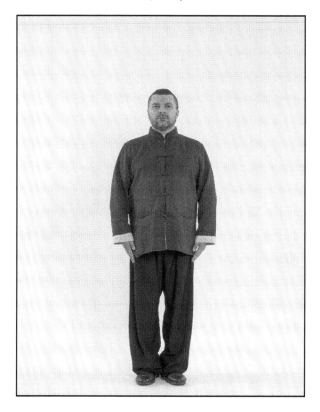

This is the first position of the form, in it we have to concentrate and perform three natural breaths, inspiring by the nose and exhaling through the nose, to achieve a state of relaxation and concentration that allows us to perform the form in a proper way.

It is of vital importance to abstract from the problems and the external distractions and to concentrate on the exercise that we are going to carry out, thus obtaining that our energy flows and is mobilized by the Meridans in a correct way.

Although it is a static posture that has no greater difficulty, its work is internal with the aim of entering a state of mental calm, looking to the east.

FIRST PALM - CHIU TIN DAAP DEI
TO THE SKY PUSHING THE EARTH

朝天踏地

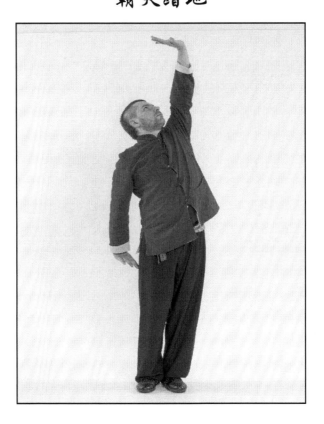

This first palm is one of the most famous exercises, several Chi Kung and Tai chi systems include it in its curriculum, such as the famous eight brocades "BAAT DYUN GAM HEI GUNG 八段錦气功".

In this exercise the circulation of energy is activated mainly of the meridians of spleen and stomach. The spleen-pancreas meridian is the Yin polarity of the earth element, the Yang polarity corresponds to the meridian of the stomach.

At the physical level, a stretch of the dorsal area is performed.

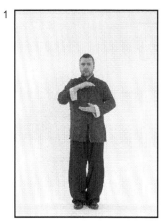 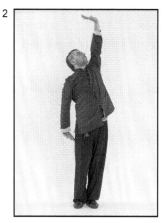
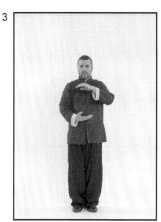 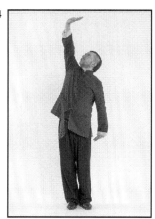

1- Take the pearl with the right hand, from the position Bei Sik we go to open the hands in a circle to catch the pearl in the center of the chest, we have to visualize that we are trapping the pearl, gathering the energy between the two palms.

2- The left hand goes up with the technique of palm DING JEUNG 頂掌, the right palm presses NGAAT 压 towards the earth. We must put our concentration on the JEUNG SAM 掌心 (center of the palm) of both hands.

3- Ditto that 1 but catching the pearl with the left hand.

4- Ditto that 2 but with the right palm towards the sky.

SECOND PALM – PAAO SAAN DOU HOI
TO REMOVE THE MOUNTAIN AND TO OVERTURN THE SEA
排山倒海

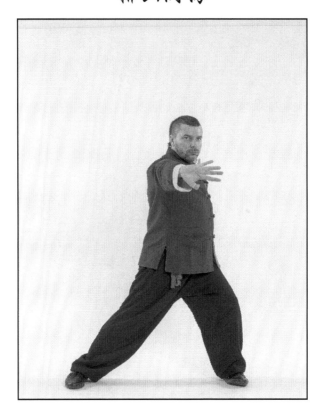

The second palm is based on one of the five animals of the Shaolin Temple 少林寺, the Dragon "LUNG".

In this exercise the circulation of energy is activated mainly in the meridians of lung and heart. The lung captures the Qi of the air, this is why so much importance is given to the good handling of the breath. The meridian of the heart is ruled by element fire is its Yin part.

At the physical level, a stretch of the Scapular area and the anterior area of the arm is performed.

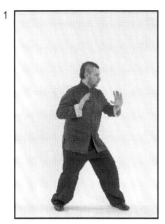
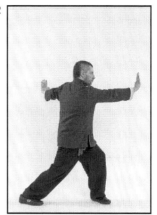
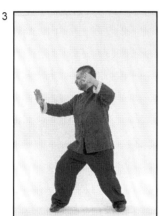
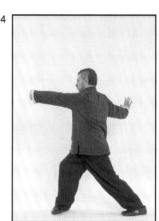

1- HOI MA 开马 Open the left foot to the north. In this movement we are in the exhalation Yin 阴 phase, all our energy is in the Low Elixir field, the HA DAAN TIN 下丹田. Hands at the level of the chest and prepared for the next stretch

2- TEUI JEUNG 推掌 push with the right hand to the north and the left hand to the back, in the DING JI MA 丁字马 posture. In this movement we are in the Yang 阳 phase.

3- Turn south, Circle with the right arm PUN KIU 蟠桥 and locate the left palm at the level of the ear SANG GUNG 生弓.

4- Push horizontally with the left palm CHAANG JEUNG 撑掌 to the south and vertically back with the right palm in the posture of DING JI MA 丁字马.

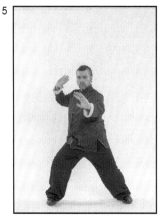
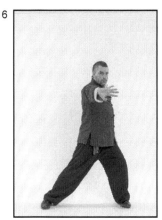
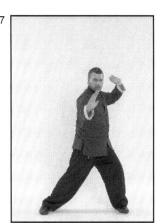
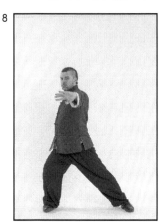

5- Circle with the left arm PUN KIU 蟠桥 and locate the right palm at the level of the ear SANG GUNG 生弓.

6- Push horizontally with the right palm CHAANG JEUNG 撑掌 to the East and vertically back with the left palm in the posture of DING JI MA 丁字马.

7- Circle with the right arm PUN KIU 蟠桥 and locate the left palm at the level of the ear SANG GUNG 生弓.

8- Push horizontally with the left palm CHAANG JEUNG 撑掌 to the east and vertically back with the right palm in the posture of DING JI MA 丁字马.

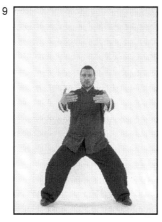
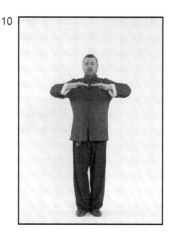
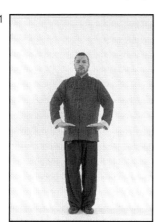
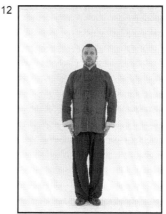

9- Both hands surround the tree JAAM JONG 站樁 in the SEI PING MA 四平马 posture.

10- Raise high the left foot SAU MA 收马 feet together HAP GEUK 合脚 placing the palms to the chest with the JEUNG SAM 掌心 towards the Earth.

11- Both palms hold the earth SEUNG HA CHAANG YUT JEUNG 双下撐月掌.

12- Relax both hands placing them to the sides SEUNG SEUI SAU 双垂手, going back to the BEI SIK 备式 posture, taking our energy to the Low Elixir Field, HA DAAN TIN 下丹田.

THIRD PALM - HAAK FU TEUI SAAN
THE BLACK TIGER PUSHES THE MOUNTAIN
黑虎推山

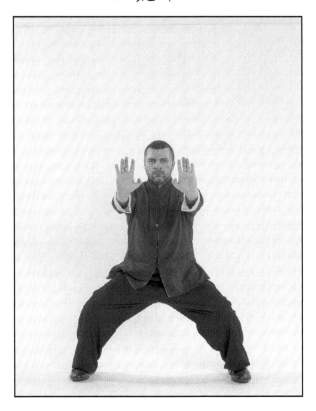

The third palm is based in other of the five animals of the Shaolin Temple 少林寺, the "FU Tiger 虎"

This exercise activates the circulation of the energy, mostly from the kidney and bladder meridians. The meridian of the kidney is the Yin polarity of the water element, its Yang polarity is the meridian of the bladder.

At the physical level is performed a stretch of the lumbar area and the back of the leg in the first two stretches activating the Yin meridians of the legs, by performing the double thrust we have to arch the back to perform a scapular stretch and the dorsal area.

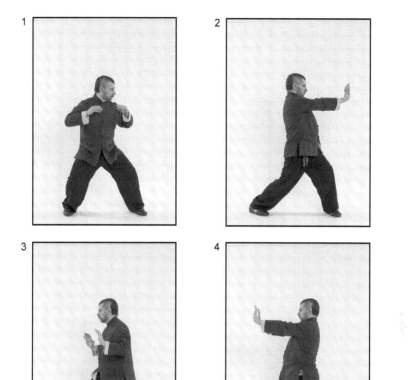

1- HOI MA 开马 Open the left foot to the north. In this movement we are in the exhalation Yin 阴 phase, all our energy is in the Low Elixir field, the HA DAAN TIN 下丹田. Hands at the level of the chest and prepared for the next stretch

2- Double push to the north while straightening the back SEUNG TEUI JEUNG 双推掌 in the DING JI MA 丁字马 posture. In this movement we are in the Yang 阳 inspiration phase.

3- Turn to the south, place the hands to the chest height prepared for the next stretch.

4- Double push to the south while straightening the back SEUNG TEUI JEUNG 双推掌 in the DING JI MA 丁字马 posture.

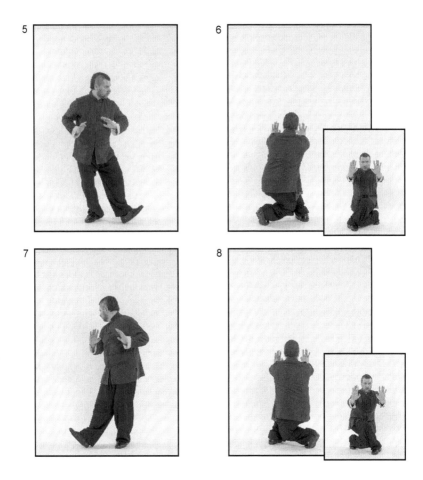

5- Turn to the north, hands at the chest level prepared for the next stretch and roll the silk with the left foot CHIN SI MA 缠丝马.

6- Finish the CHIN SI MA 缠丝马 in the DAI NAU Ma 低扭马 posture to make the double thrust directed to the South SEUNG TEUI JEUNG 双推掌.

7- Turn to the south, hands at the chest level prepared for the next stretch and roll the silk with the left foot CHIN SI MA 缠丝马.

8- Finish the CHIN SI MA 缠丝马 in the DAI NAU MA 低扭马 posture to make the double thrust directed to the South SEUNG TEUI JEUNG 双推掌.

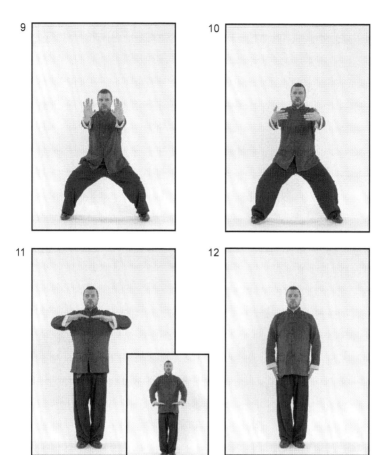

9- Turn the body to the east, open the left foot to the posture of SEI PING MA 四平马, and push with the two palms of the hands to the front SEUNG TEUI JEUNG 双推掌.

10- Both hands hug the tree JAM JOONG 站桩 in the SEI PING MA 四平马 posture.

11- Raise high the left foot SAU MA 收马 feet together HAP GEUK 合脚 placing palms of the hand to the chest with the JEUNG SAM 掌心 towards the earth, the two palms hold the earth SEUNG HA CHAANG YUT JEUNG 双下撑月掌.

12- Relax both hands placing them to the sides SEUNG SEUI SAU 双垂手, going back to the BEI SIK 备式 posture, taking our energy to the Low Elixir Field, HA DAAN TIN 下丹田.

FOURTH PALM – DAAI PAANG JIN CHI
THE SACRED GREAT BIRD OPENS HIS WINGS

大鵬展翅

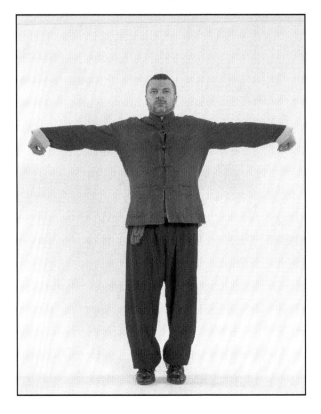

The fourth palm is based in one of the animals from the Chinese mythology, the great bird "DAAI PAANG 大鵬 (da peng in mandarin)".

This exercise activates the circulation of the energy mostly from the lung and large intestine meridians. The element of the lung is the metal in its polarity Yin, the Yang polarity is found in the meridian of the large intestine.

At the physical level, is performed a stretching of the ligaments, musculature and it gets rid of tensions from the spine, as well as a work of equilibrium is performed.

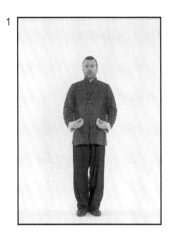
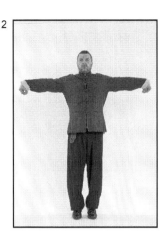

1- Staying on posture of feet together HAP GEUK 合腳 form the crane peak HOK JEUI 鶴咀.

2- Raise both arms at the same time that one of these lateral stretchings towards the north and the south is being performed, trying to touch with the crane peak the anterior part of the arm. While the arms are being raised high the ankles must be raised high until the tip toe position.

DAAI PAANG 大鵬

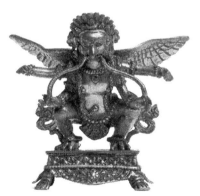

Now, what wanders free and easy is clearly the mind of the enlightened man. The Master Chuang spoke of the great Tao and expressed his meaning with the quail and the great bird Peng. Due the path of the Paang bird through life is powerful, it neglects spiritual satisfaction beyond the body. Due the quail is near, she laughs at what is distant and is happy with herself in her heart. The Enlightened Man directly ascends to heaven and joyfully wanders endlessly in freedom.

Buddhist monk Ji Deun 支遁 (350 d.C.)

FIFTH PALM – TUNG JI BAAI GUN YAM
THE KID PRAISES THE GUN YAM GODDESS
童子拜观音

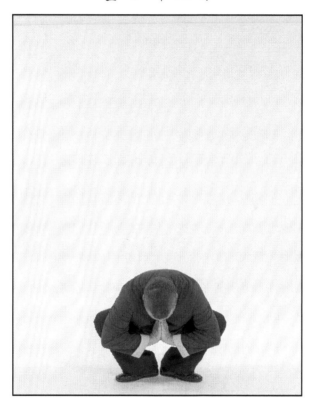

The fifth palm is dedicated to show respect for the Buddhist tradition of the Shaolin Temple 少林寺, performing the three reverences to the goddess Gun Yam 观音 (in mandarin Guan Yin).

In this exercise the circulation of energy is activated mostly for the meridians of Du Mo, kidney and bladder. The meridian Du Mai governs all Yang meridians.

On the physical level the first starts from the greeting while crouching, it performs a relaxation of the lumbar vertebrae by opening the intervertebral space, the second part of the exercise execute a stretch of all back and back area of the legs.

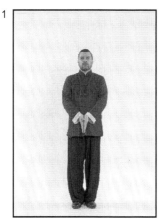
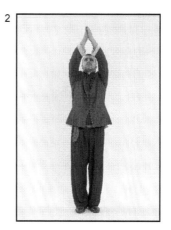
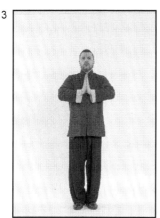
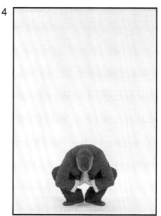

1- Opening the palms from the top till the abdomen TOU BOU 肚部, clasping the palms of the hands HAP JEUNG 合掌.

2- Move the palms to the sky TIN 天.

3- Go down till the chest HUNG BOU 胸部, in FAT JEUNG 佛掌 position (first reverence).

4- Crouch down as if you were praying squatting and bowing to the Buddha BAAI FAT SIK 拜佛式 (second reverence).

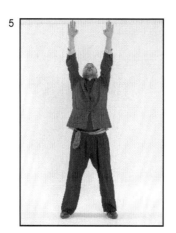
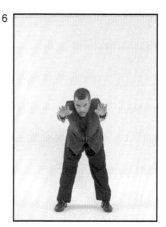
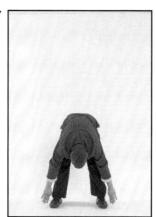

5- Then slowly get up until completely standing up and open your left foot to the SAT MA 实马 posture, and move your palms to place them on top of your head with your arms stretched.

6- Bend forward while stretching, trying to reach very far with the fingertips.

7- Move the palms till the earth DEI 地 (third reverence).

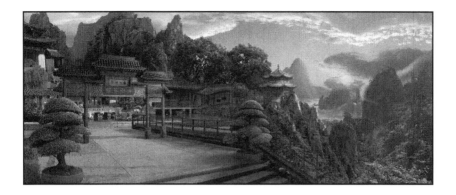

The Shaolin Monastery, founded in the year 495 A.D. is located in the middle of a big forest, near the Shao Shi (少室) hill, that's why it was granted with the name of "Shaolin Temple" (林 lin means forest in Chinese).

During the sixth century of our era, a Hindu monk, Bodhidarma 菩提达摩 (Da Mo 达摩 in Chinese), the 36th Patriarch of Mahayana Buddhism takes to Shaolin the three sutras (Tripitaka).

He was the founder of the Chan Buddhism, later known as Zen in Japan.

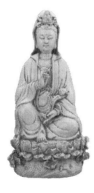

GUN YAM 观音

The name Gun Yam (Guan Yin in Mandarin) is a contraction of Guan Shi Yin 观世音, which means "who listens the sorrows of the world", is the bodhisattva of compassion.

In Taoist mythology, is known as Ci Hang Zhen Ren 慈航真人 the taoist goddess of mercy and is considered an immortal.

In popular devotion, Guanyin rescues those who come to her in times of difficulty, especially In front of the dangers caused by water, fire or weapons. The Bodhisattva understands the feelings of fear and responds to requests for help with her compassion. As a merciful mother, she hears the requests of those who wish to have children.

SIXTH PALM - SEUNG HA LAAU JAAU
FISHING IN THE BOTTOM WITH THE CLAWS
双下捞爪

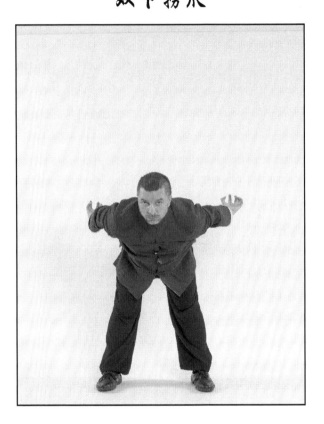

The sixth palm is based on the "FU 虎" Tiger.

In this exercise the circulation of energy is activated mostly for the meridians of Ren Mo. The Ren Mai meridian regulates the body's yin energy and has yin polarity, its yang par is the meridian Du Mai.

In a physical level, a stretch of the back of the legs is performed by activating the Yin Meridians as well as the pectoral area through the activation in the area of the shoulder's fold, where the yin meridians (pericardium, heart and lung) flow through the inner surface of the arm from the chest to the hands.

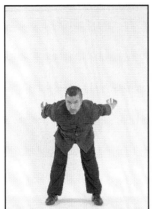
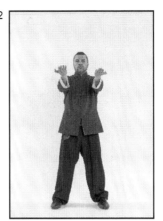
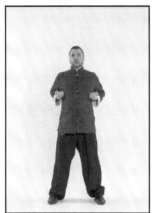

1- Take the two claws SEUNG JAAU 双爪 from down to the top, till the level of the shoulders, looking forward.

2- Stand up with your palms facing the sky with your arms outstretched.

3-, And close the fists taking them to the chest SEUNG CHUNG JONG 双冲撞, with the forearms parallel to the ground.

SEVENTH PALM – YAP JAAU AU JUNG
GREETING WITH THE CLAW IN THE CHEST
揖爪勾胸

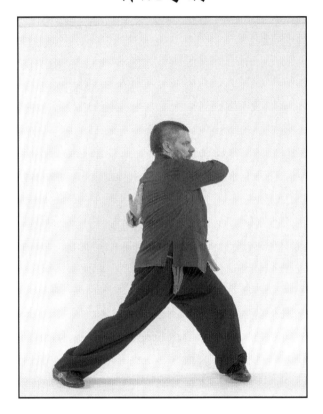

The seventh palm is based in one of the five animals of the Shaolin temple 少林寺, The Serpent "is 蛇".

In this exercise the circulation of energy is activated mostly in the Yin meridians (pericardium, heart and lung) flowing through the inner surface of the arm from the chest to the hands.

In the physical level a stretching is executed in the scapular zone that corresponds with the hand that is touching the shoulder fold.

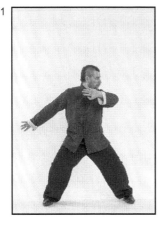
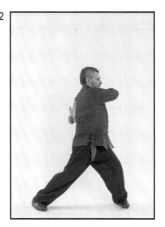
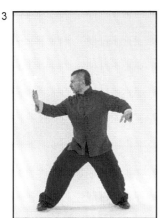
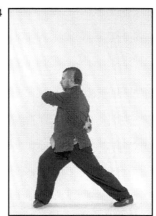

1- HOI MA 开马 Open the left foot to the north, prepare the left hand to execute the grabbing and leave extended to the back the right hand.

2- Grab NAK KIU 扚桥 and place to the chest the area of the fold of the shoulder, touching it with the back of the right palm, the left palm touches with its dorsum the back trying to place it as high as possible, in the posture of DING JI MA 丁字马.

3- Turn to the south, prepare the right hand to hold the grip and leave the left hand extended behind.

4- Grab NAK KIU 扚桥 and place to the chest the area of the fold of the shoulder, touching it with the dorsum of the left palm, the right palm touches it with the back the rear trying to carry it as high as possible, in the posture of DING JI MA 丁字马.

EIGHTH PALM - WAAN GUNG HOI GAAK
To tense the arc opening the diaphragm
挽弓开膈

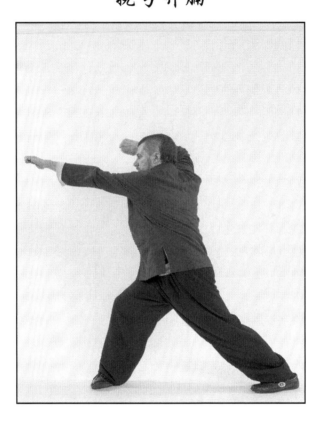

The eighth palm is one of the most famous exercises along with the first palm, that several systems of Chi Kung and Tai Chi include it in their curriculum, such as the famous eight brocades "BAAT DYUN GAM HEI GUNG 八段錦气功", with the peculiarity that we find it here executed with back torsion.

In this exercise is activated the circulation of energy mostly in the lung and large intestine meridians; it balances the lungs and the large intestine along with the meridian of the heart and the small intestine.

In the physical level a stretch of the corresponding Scapular area is performed with the hand that releases the arrow, as well as a back torsion that stretches the muscles chains that intersect in the back.

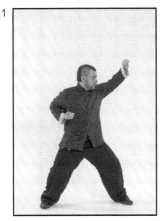
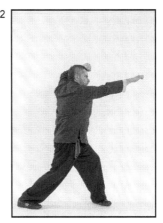
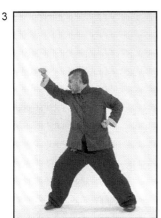
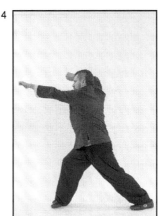

1- Turn to the north, block with the left arm GUNG KIU 攻桥.

2- Change to protect the head with the left arm and stretch the arm by releasing the fist as if it was an arrow JIN CHEUI 箭槌, in the DING JI MA 丁字马 posture.

3- Turn to the north, block with the right arm GUNG KIU 攻桥.

4- Change to protect the head with the right arm and stretch the arm throwing the fist as if it was an arrow JIN CHEUI 箭槌, in the DING JI MA 丁字马 posture.

NINTH PALM – GAM PAAU LOU JAAU
The golden leopard shows his claws
金豹露爪

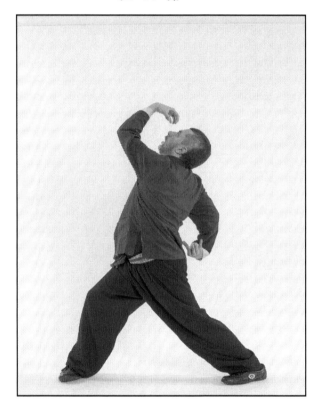

The ninth palm is based on one of the five animals of the Shaolin temple 少林寺, the Leopard "PAAU 豹".

In this exercise the circulation of energy is activated mostly in the cosmic micro orbit.

In a physical level, a stretch is performed based on the torsion of the back along with the elevation of the elbow.

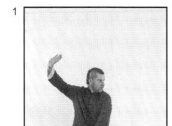
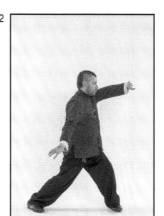
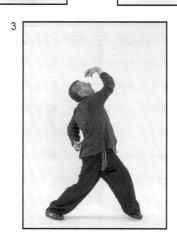

1- Turn north in the SEI PING MA 四平马 posture and prepare the palms to begin the stretch, with the left hand in the Low elixir field HA DAAN TIN 下丹田 and the right hand back to the level of the head.

2- Move by drawing a circle with your hands, raising your left hand at the level of your shoulder and your right hand at the level of your waist.

3-, To the north, form the right claw FU JAAU 虎爪 and raise it up until placing it above the mouth while is open, pulling the elbow upward, put the left claw JAAU 爪 back in line with the right claw and the mouth, in the posture of DING JI MA 丁字马. Open the mouth slightly.

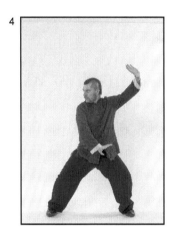
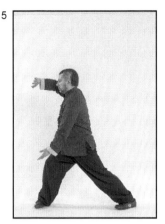
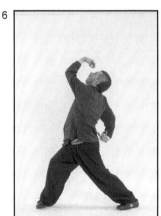

4- Turn south in the posture of SEI PING MA 四平马 and prepare the palms to begin the stretch, with the right hand In the Low elixir field HA DAAN TIN 下丹田 and the left hand back to the level of the head.

5- Move by drawing a circle with your hands, raising your right hand at the level of your shoulder and your left hand at the level of your waist.

6-, To the south, form the right claw FU JAAU 虎爪 and raise it up until placing it above the mouth while is open, pulling the elbow upward, put the right claw JAAU 爪 back in line with the left claw and the mouth, in the posture of DING JI MA 丁字马. Open the mouth slightly.

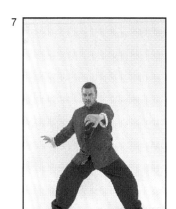
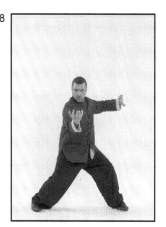
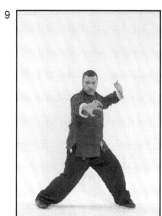

7- Turn east in the posture of SEI PING MA 四平马 and prepare the palms to begin the stretch, with the left hand in the Low elixir field HA DAAN TIN 下丹田 and the right hand back to the level of the head.

8- Move by drawing a circle with your hands, raising your left hand at the level of your shoulder and your right hand at the level of your waist.

9-, To the east, form the right claw FU JAAU 虎爪 and raise it up until placing it above the mouth while is open, pulling the elbow upward, put the left claw JAAU 爪 back in line with the right claw and the mouth, in the posture of DING JI MA 丁字马. Open the mouth slightly.

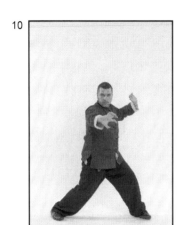
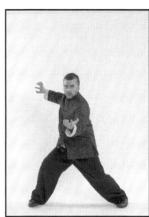
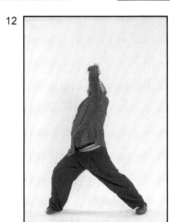

10- Turn east in the posture of SEI PING MA 四平马 and prepare the palms to begin the stretch, with the right hand in the Low elixir field HA DAAN TIN 下丹田 and the left hand back to the level of the head.

11- Move by drawing a circle with your hands, raising your right hand at the level of your shoulder and your left hand at the level of your waist.

12-, To the east, form the right claw FU JAAU 虎爪 and raise it up until placing it above the mouth while is open, pulling the elbow upward, put the right claw JAAU 爪 back in line with the right claw and the mouth, in the posture of DING JI MA 丁字马. Open the mouth slightly.

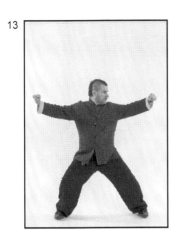
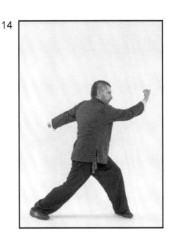

13- Turn north, circle with the left palm PUN KIU 蟠桥 in the posture of SEI PING MA 四平马 and close both.fists.

14- Throw slowly a long hook with the right fist FAAN JONG 反撞 while stretching towards the north, in the posture of DING JI MA 丁字马.

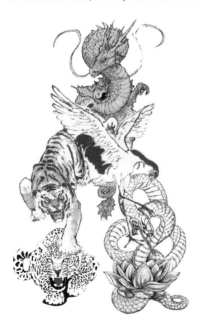

SIU LAM NG YING 少林五形

The five Siu Lam (Shaolin) animals are present in the next form.

We find Lung 龙 (Dragon) who cultivates the Shen (spirit), with Fu 虎 (Tiger) who strengthens bones and muscles, Paau 豹 (Leopard) who increases the vigor and the power, Se 蛇 (serpent) who activates the Qi (vital energy) and Hok 鹤 (Crane) who preserves the Jing (essence).

During the Song Dynasty 宋朝 (960-1278 A.D.) Gok Yun 觉元, Lei Sau 李德 and Baak Yuk Fung 白玉峯 developed the form of the five animals, which contributed to completing the new Siu Lam system.

TENTH PALM - TEUI LIK DONG DIT
TO KICK WITH THE BALANCING ENERGY

腿力蕩跌

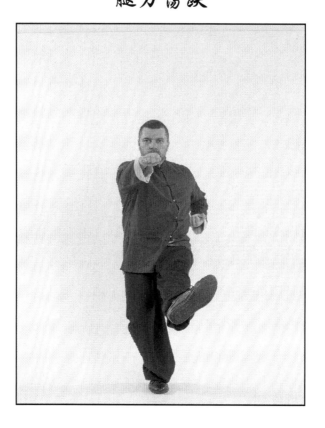

The tenth palm is based on the mythological animal Golden Rooster "FUNG WONG 凤凰 (Feng Huang in Mandarin)".

In this exercise is activated the circulation of energy mosty for the bladder and small intestine meridians, the Qi is mobilized downward and it concentrates in the low elixir field HA DAAN TIN 下丹田. The meridian of the small intestine belongs to the element fire, through its internal route, from the spot 18 the energy flows to the spot 1 of the meridian of the bladder, is the Yang channel of the element water.

At the physical level, is performed a stretch of the posterior part of the leg and the work of the balance, as well as a back torsion that stretches the muscular chains that intersect in the back.

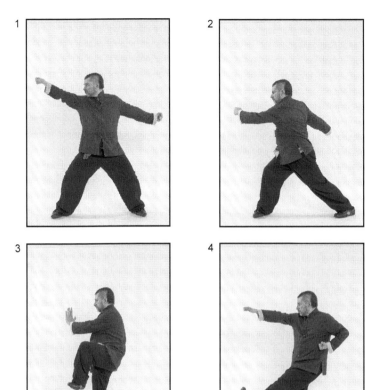

1- Turn south move your right arm in a top-bottom circle GWA CHEUI 挂槌.

2- The left arm also describes a circle from the top to the bottom KAP CHEUI 扱槌.

3- Circle with the left palm PUN KIU 蟠桥.

4- Left kick CHAANG GEUK 撑脚 slowly executed in stretch, at the same time release the right fist CHEUNG NGAAM CHEUI 抡眼槌 while slowly stretching, standing in the posture of one leg DUK GEUK 独脚.

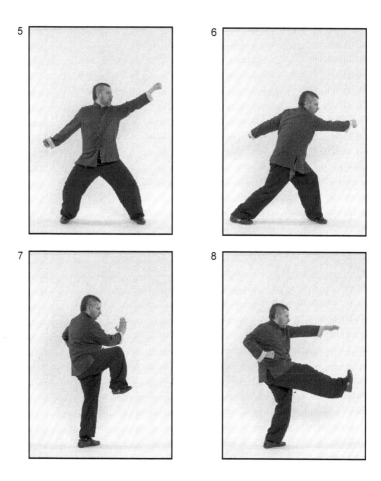

5- Turn north move your left arm in a top-bottom circle GWA CHEUI 挂槌.

6- The right arm also describes a circle from the top to the bottom KAP CHEUI 扱槌.

7- Circle with the right palm PUN KIU 蟠桥.

4- Right kick CHAANG GEUK 撐脚 slowly executed in stretch, at the same time release the left fist CHEUNG NGAAM CHEUI 抡眼槌 while slowly stretching, standing in the posture of one leg DUK GEUK 独脚.

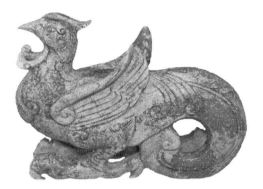

FUNG WONG 鳳鳳

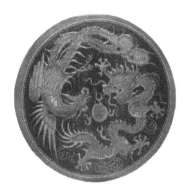

Is a mythological bird of East Asia that reigns over all birds. Originally the males were called Feng and the females Huang, but such distinction was left behind and became a unique female entity that is matched with the Chinese dragon, which is considered masculine.

The typical image of the fenghuang protrayed him attacking snakes with his heels and wings extended. According to the chapter 17 Shiniao of the Erya encyclopedia, the Fenghuang is composed of the rooster's beak and forehead, the face of a swallow, neck of serpent, goose chest, back of turtle, hind quarters of a deer and the tail of a fish.

His body symbolizes the six celestial bodies. The head is the sky, the eyes are the sun, the back is the moon, the wings are the wind, the feet are the earth and the tail represents the planets. Its feathers contain the five fundamental colors: black, white, red, green and yellow.

During the Han Dynasty, 2200 years ago, two birds one male (Feng 鳳) and another female (Huang 鳳) were seen looking at each other. Then, during the Yuan dynasty, the two terms were combined to become Fenghuang, being the "King of the Birds" the symbol of the empress when she was paired with the dragon, as it was the symbol of the emperor. The Fung Wong represented the power sent to the Empress by the heavens.

ELEVENTH PALM – YI SAAN DOU HOI
TO MOVE THE MOUNTAIN AND TO OVERTURN THE SEA
移山倒海

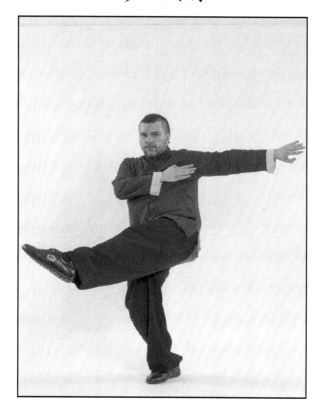

The eleventh palm is based on one of the five animals of the Shaolin temple 少林寺, the Leopard "PAAU 豹".

In this exercise the circulation of energy is activated mostly of the gallbladder meridian. The meridian of the gallbladder is the yang part of the wood element.

In the physical level, a stretch of the abdominal belt is executed, along with the external side of the leg, as well as a back torsion.

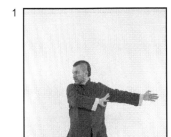
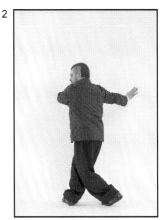
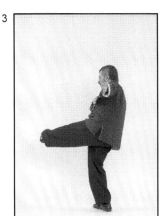

1- Put down the right foot to the back in the SEI PING MA 四平马 posture, opening the arms to the north.

2- Curl up in the NAU MA 扭马 position, move at the same time the arms towards the West drawing a circle above the head.

3- Perform a sweep towards the west with the left leg stretched SOU GEUK 扫脚 stretch slowly and at the same time in the opposite direction place the arms extended from right to left SEUNG BUT KIU 双拔桥.

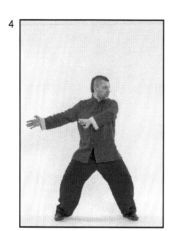
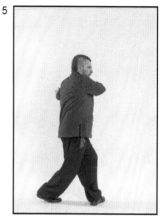
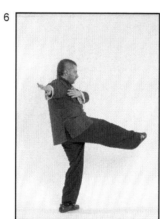

4- Put down the right foot to the back in the SEI PING MA 四平马 posture, opening the arms to the south.

5- Curl up in the NAU MA 扭马 position, move at the same time the arms towards the West drawing a circle above the head.

6- Perform a sweep towards the west with the left leg stretched SOU GEUK 扫脚 stretch slowly and at the same time in the opposite direction place the arms extended from left to right SEUNG BUT KIU 双拨桥.

The dragon pearl - LUNG JYU 龙珠

He lived on the island of Borneo, on the highest mountain of the Kinabalu Island, a peaceful dragon that passionately guarded a precious pearl. Every day he played with it; He threw it into the air and picked it up with his mouth. He felt delightful with his exquisite pearl and never asked anything more to his days. Many had vainly tried to steal his treasure, because the dragon was not willing to lose his only possession.

However, the emperor of China was willing to challenge the Pacific Dragon, so he requested his firstborn, the hair of the crown, to get the pearl for the imperial treasure. After several days of voyage, the Prince spotted the mountain and, at its peak, he saw the playful dragon. He developed a plan to snatch his pearl without any danger. He ordered his men to build a kite capable enough to support the weight of a man and a paper lantern.

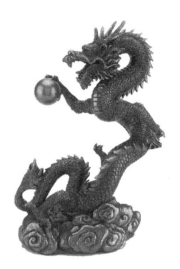

After seven days of hard work, the Prince's men finished the kite, the most beautiful ever seen. At nightfall, he stood on the kite and flew up to the top of the mountain.

He slowly got inside of the cave. The dragon was sleeping with any worry, carrying the precious pearl on its legs. With great care, he snatched the jewel and instead left the paper lantern. He signaled his men to pick up the kite rope. He landed, safe and sound, on the boat.

When the dragon woke up, he discovered that someone took the pearl away from him, leaving him a paper lantern. He burst in rage. He began to fire and smoke through his mouth and threw himself down the hill to catch the thieves. He traced every corner of the island, until he saw a Chinese junk on the high seas. He rushed to the ship and shouted with all his might, "Give me my pearl back!" The sailors were terrified.

The prince, in a desperate attempt to escape from the Dragon, commanded the largest cannon and fired at his furious pursuer. The Dragon saw a ball coming out of the powder cloud and thought it was his pearl. He opened his mouth to collect his jewel, and sank into the depths of the sea. The prince and his men returned triumphant, and the pearl became the most precious jewel in the kingdom of China.

TWELFTH PALM - YAU JEUN LUNG TAAM HOI
THE GREAT DRAGON SEARCHES IN THE SEA
右骏龙探海

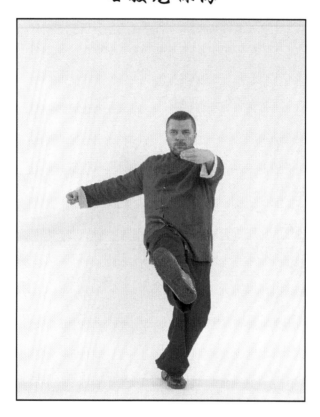

The twelfth palm appears two of the five animals of the Shaolin temple 少林寺, the Crane and the Dragon "HOK 鹤 LUNG 龙". In this part the Dragon takes the pearl with the right claw.

In this exercise with the kick WAANG CHAANG GEUK 横撑脚 we work the energy of stomach meridian that is associated with the Earth element and represents its yang polarity. With the CHAANG GEUK 撑脚 kick is the same work as in the tenth palm and with the kick DA GEUK 打脚 we work the energy of the bladder meridian.

In the physical level a stretch of the right leg and a great work of balance are performed, as well as a back torsion that stretches the muscle chains that intersect in the back.

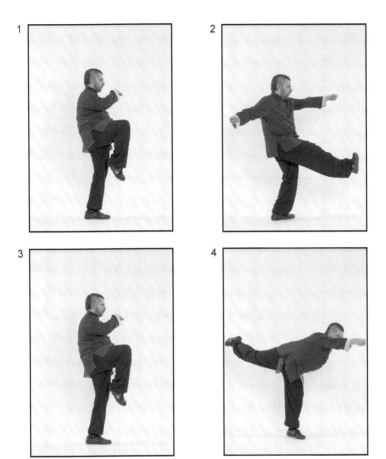

1- Lift the horse HEI MA 起马 and stay in the DUK GEUK 独脚 posture, take the pearl JYU LUNG 珠龙 with the right arm.

2- Kick to the front CHAANG GEUK 撑脚 slowly executed while stretching, at the same time close the hands with crane's beak shape HOK JEUI 鹤咀, the left beak to the south and the right beak to the back.

3- Back to the DUK GEUK 独脚 posture, take the pearl JYU LUNG 珠龙 with your right arm.

4- Crouch forward and right side kick backwards WAANG CHAANG GEUK 横撑脚 slowly executed while stretching, at the same time they close HOK JEUI 鹤咀, the right beak to the south and the left peak backward.

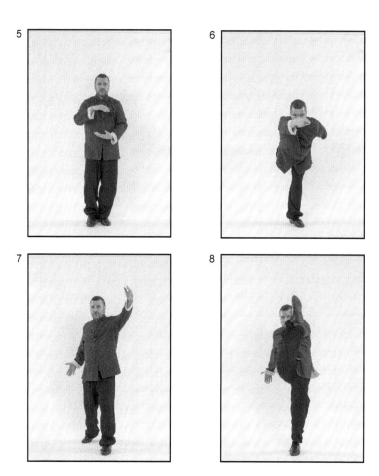

5- Pick up the right leg turn the body to the east with your feet together HAP GEUK 合脚, take the pearl JYU LUNG 球龙 with your right arm.

6- Crouch forward and right side kick backwards WAANG CHAANG GEUK 横撑脚 slowly executed while stretching, at the same time they close HOK JEUI 鹤咀, the right beak to the east and the left peak backward.

7- Lower your right leg to the ground open your arms with the right arm to the back and down and the left arm to the east and up.

8- Right kick gives DA GEUK 打脚 to the east executed quickly and explosively, use the left hand to hit on the back of the right foot.

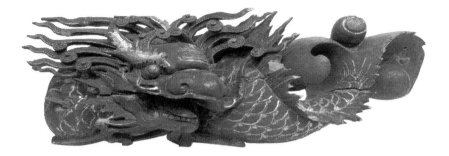

THE DRAGON - LUNG 龙

The first legendary emperor of China, used a snake in his coat of arms. Every time he conquered a new tribe he incorporated the emblem of the defeated enemy into his emblem. This explains why the dragon seems to have different characteristics of other animals.

For the Han Dynasty the appearance of the Dragon was described as a being with the trunk of a serpent, the scales of a carp, the tail of a whale, the horns of a deer, the face of a camel, the claws of an eagle, the ears of a bull, the feet of a tiger and the eyes of a lobster, besides of having a flaming pearl under his chin.

Chinese dragons are strongly water-related in popular beliefs. They are believed to be the rulers of the moving water bodies, such as waterfalls, rivers and seas. There are four main Dragon Kings, representing each of the four seas: The East, South, West and North Sea.

It is said that the legendary first emperor Huang Di was immortalized as a dragon that resembled his emblem and ascended to heaven. Because the Chinese consider Huang Di as their ancestor, they sometimes call themselves "The Descendants of the Dragon."

There are "Nine Classic Types" of Dragons: Tianlong (天龙) The Celestial Dragon, Shenlong (神龙) The Spiritual Dragon, Fucanglong (伏藏龙) The Dragon of Hidden Treasures, Dilong (地龙) The Dragon of the Underworld, Yinglong (应龙) The Winged Dragon, Jiaolong (虬龙) The Horned Dragon, Palong (蟠龙) The Curled Dragon, which inhabits the waters, Huanglong (黄龙) The Yellow Dragon, which emerged from the Luo River to teach Fuxi the elements of Scripture and Dragon King (龙王).

Apart from these, there are nine Dragon sons: Bixi 贔屭, Chiwen 螭吻, Pulao 蒲牢, Taotie 饕餮, Baxia 蚣蝮, Yazi 睚眦, Ananni 狻猊 and Jiaotu 椒圖. There are two other (inferior) species of dragon, the Jiao and the Li, both without horns.

THIRTEENTH PALM - YAU JEUN LUNG TAAM HOI
THE GREAT DRAGONS SEARCHES IN THE SEA
左骏龙探海

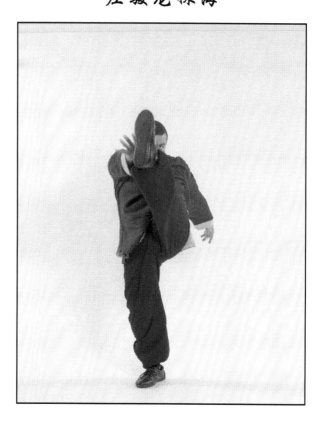

In the thirteenth palm appear two of the five animals of the Shaolin temple 少林寺, the Crane and the Dragon "HOK 鹤 LUNG 龙". In this part the Dragon takes the pearl with the left claw.

In this exercise with the kick WAANG CHAANG GEUK 横撑脚 we work the energy of the stomach meridian that is associated with the Earth element and represents its yang polarity. With the kick CHAANG GEUK 撑脚 we have the same work as in the tenth palm and with the kick DA GEUK 打脚 we work the energy of the bladder meridian.

In a physical level a stretch of the right leg and a great work of balance are performed, as well as a back torsion that stretches the muscle chains that intersect in the back.

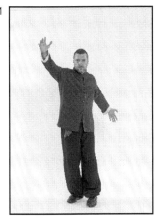 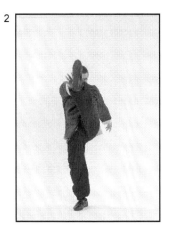

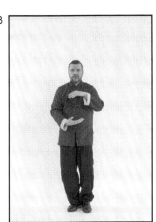 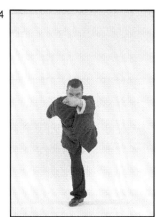

1- Lower your right leg to the ground to feet together HAP GEUK 合脚 open your arms with your left arm to the back and down and the right arm to the East and up.

2- Left kick gives DA GEUK 打脚 towards the east quickly and explosively executed, use the right hand to hit on the back of the left foot.

3- Lower your right leg to the ground to feet together HAP GEUK 合脚, grab the pearl JYU LUNG 珠龙 with the left arm.

4- Crouch forward and left side kick backwards WAANG CHAANG GEUK 横撑脚 slowly executed while stretching, at the same time they close HOK JEUI 鹤咀, the left beak to the east and the right peak backwards.

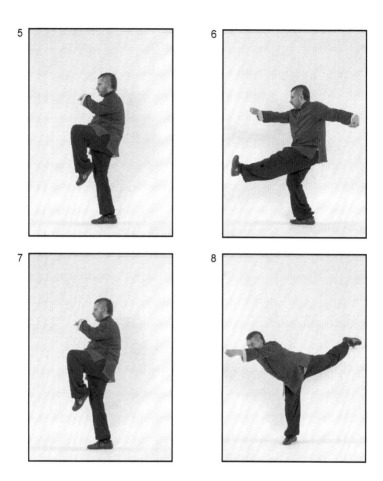

5- Lift the horse HEI MA 起马 and stay in the DUK GEUK 独脚 posture, take the pearl JYU LUNG 珠龙 with the left arm.

6- Crouch forward and left side kick backwards CHAANG GEUK 橫撐腳 slowly executed while stretching, at the same time they close HOK JEUI 鶴咀, the right beak to the north and the left peak backwards.

7- Go back to the DUK GEUK 独脚 posture; grab the pearl JYU LUNG 珠龙 with the left arm.

8- Crouch forward and right side kick backwards WAANG CHAANG GEUK 橫撐腳 slowly executed while stretching, at the same time they close HOK JEUI 鶴咀, the left beak to the north and the right peak backwards.

THE RED CROWNED CRANE - DAAN DING HOK 丹頂鶴

The red crowned Crane was the symbol of China in ancient times. In the traditional Chinese painting, the painters frequently drew the crane on their paper. Already in the spring and autumn and the period of the Warring Kingdoms (772-475 BC), the red crown of the crane is located in the bronze wares and many sacrificial cups. In Taoism, this bird represents longevity and immortality.

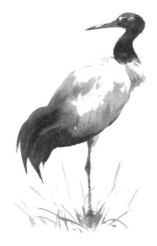

It lives in fields and high valleys with soggy areas, where the height constitutes a natural advantage, being able to have vision of the danger from a safe distance.

The flight is powerful, with the neck and legs extended, and with paused flutters, interspersed with glides.

Its average longevity is between 50 and 60 years, that's why it acquires the nickname of "Immortal Crane".

The crane is believed to be able to fly souls to heaven, and funeral processions are often placed a statue of a crane in flight on top of the coffin.

In the Chinese mythology and legends, people used to change to cranes. The mythical taoist figure TIng Ling-wei, for example, It is said that he has become into a crane after spending 1.000 years in the mountains studying taoism. The he flew to the sky as an immortal.

The guest of the cavern

They say that when Lu Yan was born, a rainbow was suspended on the roof of the house. The room was filled with a delicate perfume and it resonated with supernatural music. A white crane came through the window and alighted at the bedside to sway the mother's face. They called a fortune-teller to examine the newborn. As he felt it, he declared: Crane skull, tiger members, Dragon face, Phoenix eyes, this child is not an ordinary being. He was already among the sages in another life, and in this he will perform the Supreme Union with the Dao.

Tales of the Taoist sages, Pascal Fauliot 2006

FOURTEENTH PALM - JO AU JAAU HOI
FISHING WITH THE CLAW IN THE SEA
左勾爪海

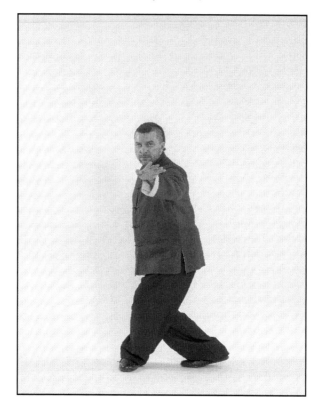

The fourteenth palm also gets the name of the Buddha walks with unbalanced steps and is based on the Buddha figure.

In this exercise it activates the circulation of energy mostlyy of the small intestine meridian, the Qi is mobilized downwards and it concentrates in the low elixir field DAAN TIN 下丹田.

In a physical level is a work of cross-steps agility and changes in weight.

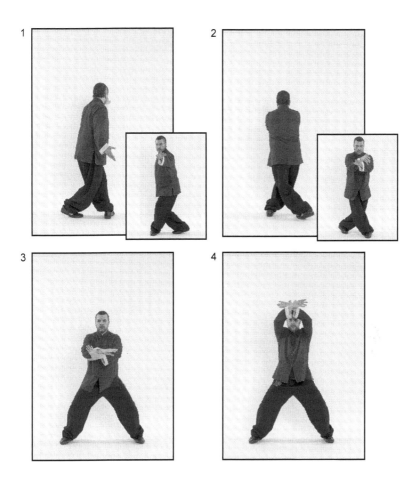

1- Turn the left foot as if you were going to rol the silk CHIN SI MA 缠丝马 to the west in the NAU MA 扭马 position and grab with the right hand LAP KIU 擸桥.

2- Step with the right foot DAAP MA 蹓马 with crossing-steps to the south, finishing in the NAU MA 扭马 position, the right hand presses over the left forearm LUK KIU 碌桥.

3- Turn the body towards the east, open the right foot to the south with the SEI PING MA 四平马 posture.

4- Open your arms in a circle while crossing them over the head SEUNG GAM JIN 上金剪.

FIFTEENTH PALM - LO HON SAAI TOU
LO HAN SHOWS HIS ABDOMEN TO THE SUN
罗汉晒肚

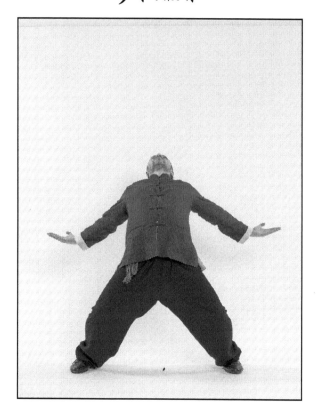

The fifteenth palm is also based on the Buddha.

In this exercise is activated the circulation of energy mostly of the Ren Mai meridian and is activated the Yin and Yang energy of the body.

In a physical level is a spine stretch, you have to stretch back at the same time you arch your back, while opening at the same time the chest and diaphragm.

1. Crouching back showing the belly and opening the arms showing the palms to the Sun SEUNG TAAT JEUNG 双挞拳.

THE BODHIDARMA MONK 菩提达摩 (DAAT MO 达摩 da mo in mandarin)

He was a monk of Hindu origin, the twenty-eighth Patriarch of Buddhism and the first legendary patriarch and founder of the form of Zen or Chan Buddhism. Coming from southern India, he arrived to China under the reign of Emperor Leung Mou Dai 梁武帝 (liang wu di in mandarin) (502-549 d. C).

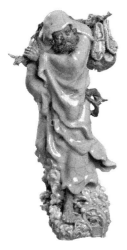

He is known as the Legitimate Master of martial arts. Before arriving In China, Da Mo had already performed three periods of intense meditation.

Da Mo was established in Shaolin to start with his teaching. To the north of the monastery, halfway to the mountain of the five animals, there is a small cave, the size of a small room, which looks directly into the sun.

Da Mo meditated in a total of nine years sitting in front of the cave in a chana state (chan meditation).

So the years went by, and when he got tired he would stand up and start exercising, he would mimic some of the movements and defense strategies of the animals he watched around him.

It is said that after spending three thousand days looking at the wall, his shadow was marked on the stone and in this you can see the figure of a man sitting with his legs crossed and his hands placed to the front together in meditation.

Outside the cave, on the west wall, is written a four-verse poem composed during the Ming dynasty by his Ming for his Minnwang of Changdan, which says:

Who can dominate the wisdom from the west?
Nine years of training in the mountain of five animals.
If the real understanding can be reached in the world of men,
Then is Da Mo who has reached that end.

When Da Mo left this world, the other monks in the Shaolin monastery, as a way to remember it, removed the wall stone where he used to meditate. And they placed it inside the monastery so that everyone could admire it.

SIXTEENTH PALM – YAU AU JAAU HOI
PESCAR CON LA GARRA EN EL MAR

右勾爪海

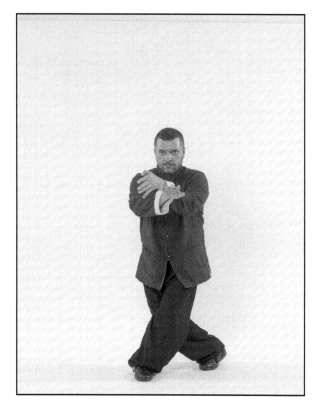

The sixteenth palm also gets the name of the Buddha walking with unbalanced steps and is based on the Buddha figure.

In this exercise is activated the circulation of energy mostly of the small intestine meridian, the Qi is mobilized downwards and it concentrates in the low elixir field HA DAAN TIN 下丹田.

In a physical level is a work of cross-steps agility and changes in weight.

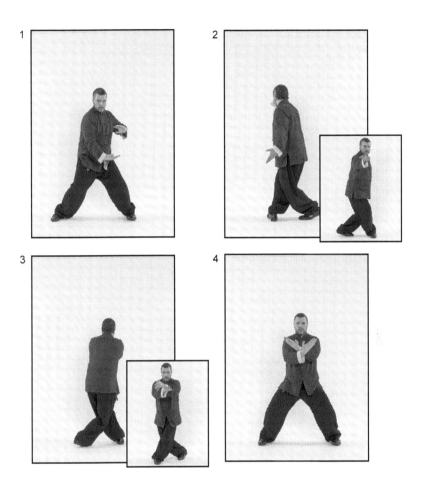

1- Slightly turn the body to the left and take the Pearl JYU LUNG 珠龙 with the left arm.

2. Turn the right foot as if you were going to roll the silk CHIN SI MA 缠丝马 to the west in the NAU MA 扭马 posture and grab with the left hand LAP KIU 攋桥.

3- Step with the right foot DAAP MA 蹭马 with crossed steps to the north, finish in the NAU MA 扭马 position, the left hand presses above the right forearm LUK KIU 碌桥.

4- Turn the body to the east, open the left foot to the north to the posture of SEI PING MA 四平马, the arms are crossed in front of the chest.

SEVENTEENTH PALM - SEUNG JIN JI
DOUBLE ARROW FINGERS
双箭指

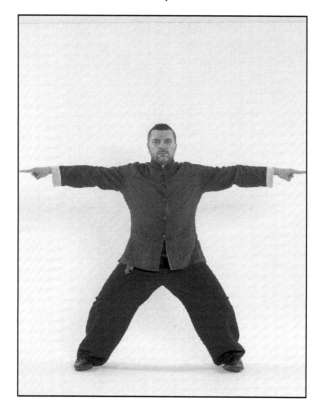

The seventeenth palm also receives the name of the Buddha points the way and is based on the figure of Buddha.

In this exercise the energy Jing 精 is stored in the low elixir field HA DAAN TIN 下丹田.

In a physical level a stretch of the dorsal is executed.

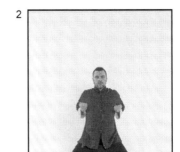

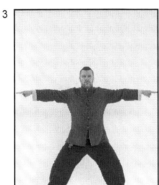

1- Keeping the SEI PING MA 四平马 posture, we lift up the fists to the waits CHUK YIU 束腰.

2- Raise the fist to your chest level SEUNG CHUNG JONG 双冲撞.

3-Stretch your arms in a parallel position to the earth, pointing with your index fingers and heart to north and south JIN JI 箭指.

EIGHTEENTH PALM - SEUNG HA CHUNG KYUN
THROW BOTH FISTS DOWN

双下冲拳

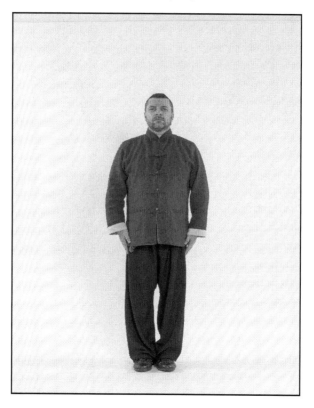

The eighteenth palm is a return to the meditative state.

The energy is raised up to Baak Wui 百会 (Bai hui in Mandarin) the highest point of the body and goes down to the low elixir field HA DAAN TIN 下丹田.

In a physical level a stretch of the arms to the sky is being performed in order to finish the form.

* Bai Hui 百会: An acupuncture point located in the upper part of the head. It is translated as "a hundred meetings". In the esoteric Daoism is also the point where numerous spirits converge and the point where Chung Mak 衝脈 (Chong Mai in Mandarin) extends upward the body.

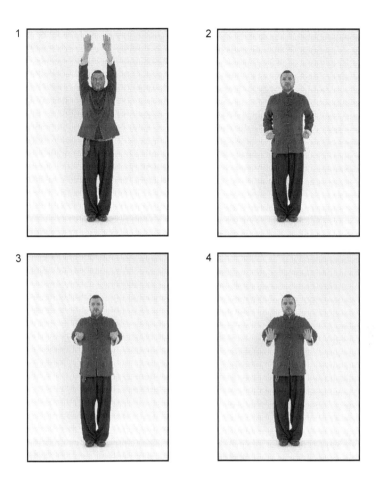

1- We lift up the left foot SAU MA 收马 to the posture of feet together HAP GEUK 合脚 and at the same time we elevate the arms in a circle until the fingers point to the sky.

2- Lower your arms straight down at the waist level, close your fists and pick them up at the waist CHUK YIU 束腰.

3- Lift your fists to your chest level SEUNG CHUNG JONG 双冲撞.

4- Open the palms towards the earth.

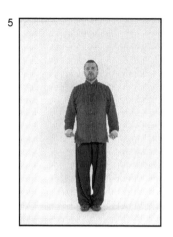 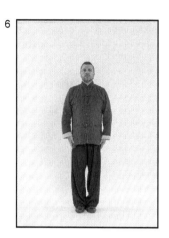

5- Push the palms to the earth until extending your arms.

6- Move to the Sau Sik 收式 posture.

Luis Lázaro Leo · 83

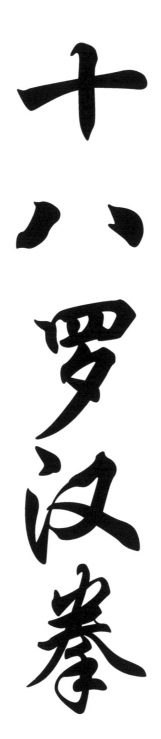

84 · CHAPTER 6

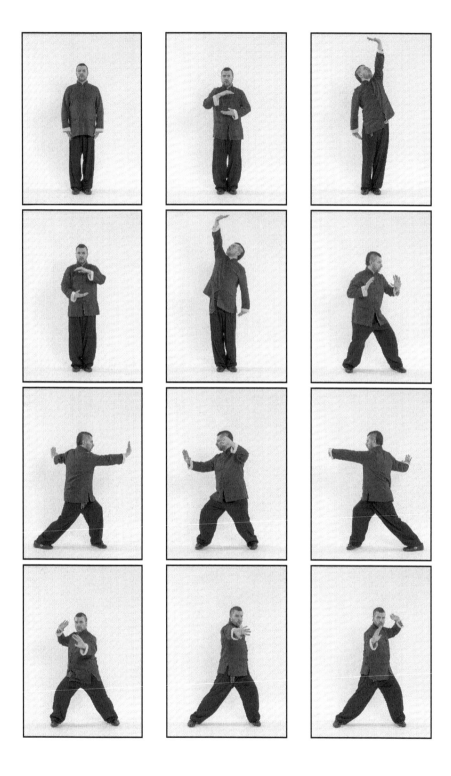

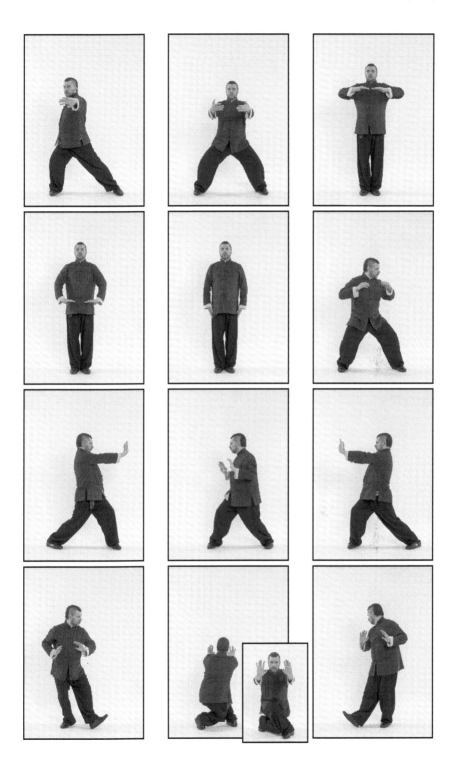

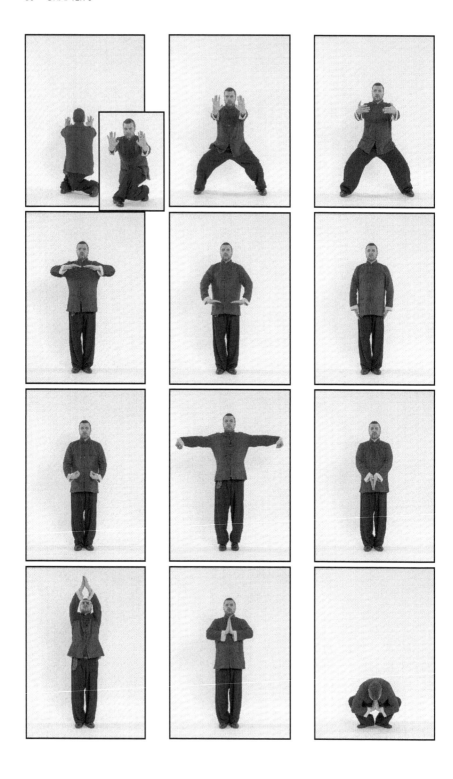

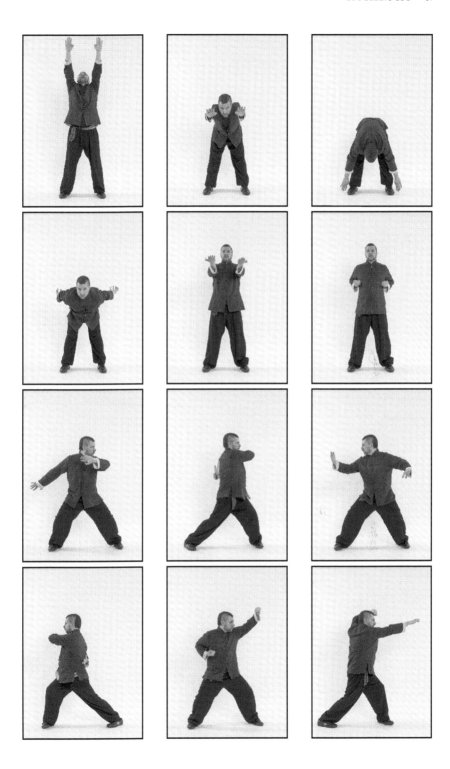

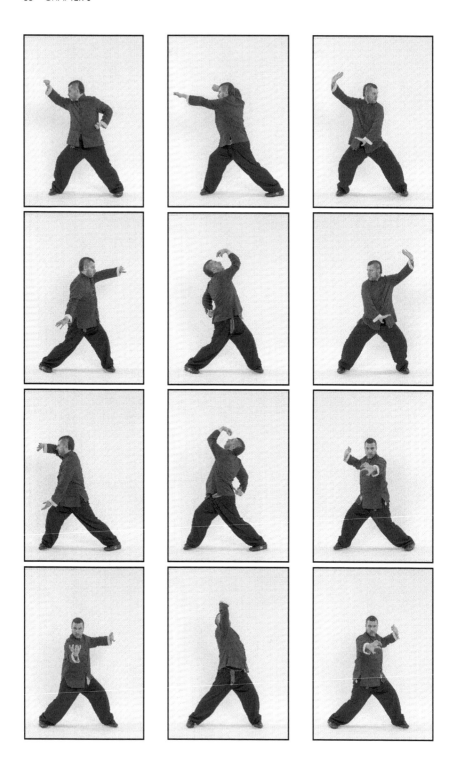

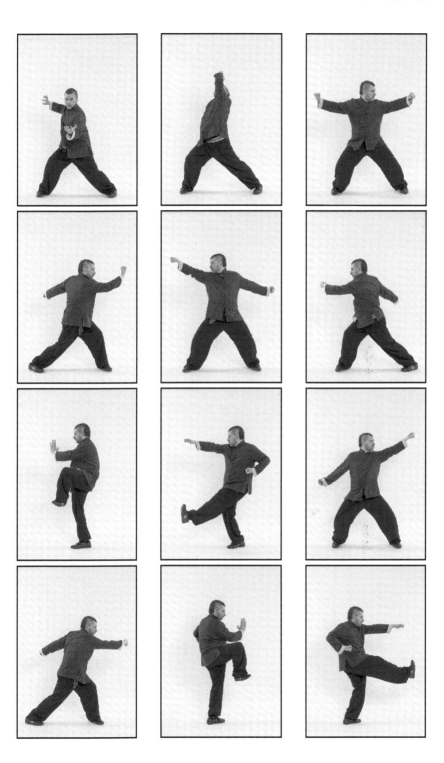

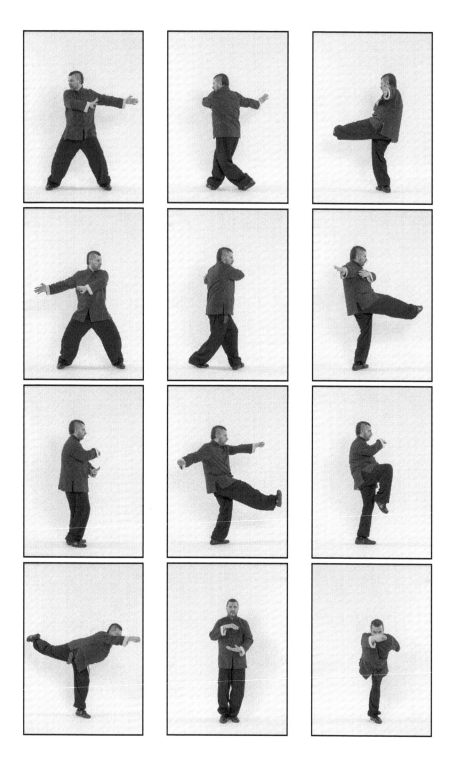

Luis Lázaro Leo · 91

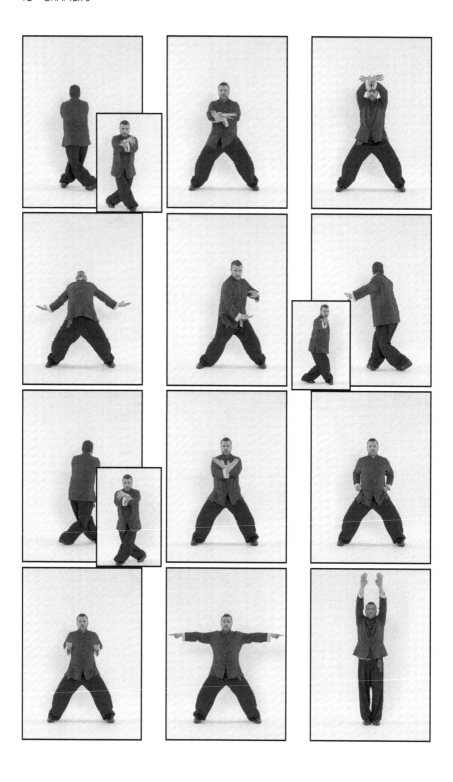

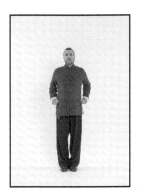 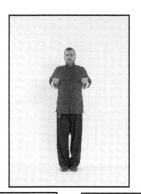 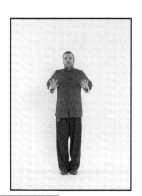
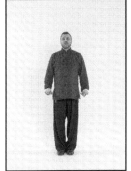 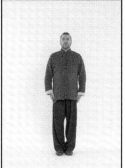

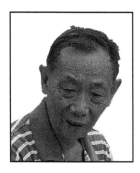

蔡李佛拳第五代传人潘顺遂先生
Pun Seun Seui 5ª generación del Choy Lee Fut

Pun Seun Seui 潘顺遂 es uno de los máximos representantes de la Familia Chan dentro de China, ya que su padre pasó a encargarse de gran parte de las escuelas de Chan Yiu Chi.

Nació el 32º año de la República de China el 15 de octubre de 1944.

While growing up, he used to train with his father, the famous masters Wong Cheung 黄昌 and the third generation of Chan Yiu Chi. Master Pun was very fortunate to be able to enhance and deepen his technique with the master Chan Yiu Chi.

After long years of training, he became his father's (Pun Fan) assistant. After the founda- tion of the General association of Choy Lee Fut in Canton province 广东省蔡李佛拳总会 and the association of Choy Lee Fut of Guang Zhou 广州市蔡李佛拳会 in the nineties, Pun Seun Seui was appointed as the Sports Director of the rst one and the head coach of the second one, where he also worked as a trainer for the advanced level.

At the same time he is the head coach of the Guang Zhou 广州技击会 ght club, and head coach in the Martial Arts national museum of Choy lee Fut Pun Fan 广州蔡李佛潘芬国术馆. He is also head coach of the Wong Cheung Club of Choy Lee Fut in Guang Zhou 广州蔡李佛 黄昌馆. He had trained many Choy Lee Fut instructors since the sixties applying the instructions given by his father Pun Fan.

He and his father had a profound friendship with the three families of Choy Lee Fut: Hung Sing 雄胜, Hung Sing 鸿胜 y Buk Sing 北胜.

A list of some of the positions Sifu Pun currently holds

- Rank 7 professional of the Chinese martial arts united
- Vice president and director of the Choy Lee Fut department in the Chinese martial arts united of Canton province.
- Honorary president of the department Choy Lee Fut in the Chinese martial arts united of Guang Zhou city - Vice-president of the department of Choy Lee Fut in the martial art united of Guang Zhou city
- Director of the Pun Fan of martial arts academy of Choy Lee Fut in Guang Zhou city
- President of the Brotherhood of Pun Fan of Choy Lee Fut in Guang Zhou
- Director of the Wong Cheung academy 黄昌 of Choy Lee Fut in Guang Zhou
- Vice-president of the oldest academy of Chan Heung, founder of Choy Lee Fut .
- Honorable president of the alliance for the commemoration of Chan Heung founder of Choy Lee Fut
- Honorable president of Choy Lee Fut international union.
- Honorable president of San Wui 新会 founder union.
- Distinguished director of Hung Sing 鸿胜 academy, the oldest of Fo Shan,
- Honorable president of the CHoy Lee Fut Alliance of USA.
- Honorable president of the Dragon and Tiger Group from the Sing Yi 胜义 acedemy of Choy Lee Fut of Vietnam

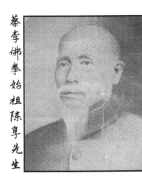

Chan Heung founder of Choy Lee Fut

He was also known as Chan Din Ying 陈典英 or Daat Ting 达庭.

He was born on July 10, 1815 During the Ching dynasty 清朝 on the 19th year of the emperor Ga Hing 嘉庆皇帝 (year of the pig).

He died on October 20, 1881 at the age of 66. During the sixth year of the emperor Gwong Seui 光绪皇帝.

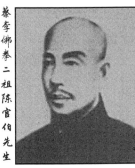

Chan Gun Baak 2nd Generation of Chey Lee Fut

Syun Gang 孙庚 was his name, Chan Heung's second son.

He was born on July 21, 1851. During the Ching Dynasty on the first year of the emperor Haam Fung 咸丰 (year of the snake)

He died on January 28, 1916, at the age of 60. During the 5th year of the Republic of China.

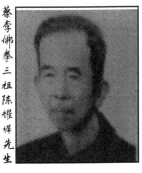

Chan Yiu Chi 3rd generation of Choy Lee Fut

Chan Yiu Chi 陈耀墀 whose title is Mau Jung 谋颂, also known as Chan Nga Wong 陈亚旺, he was Chan Gun Baak's 陈官伯 second son.

He was born on December 13, 1888. During the Ching dynasty on the 13th year of the emperor Gwong Seiu (year of the dragon)

He died on July 5, 1965 at the age of 73.

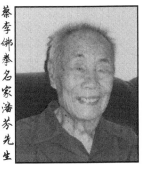

Pun Fan 4th generation of Choy Lee Fut

Pun Fan 潘芬 is a famous master and disciple of the great master Chan Yiu Chi.

He was born on November 21, 1904 during the Ching dynasty on the 29th year of the emperor Gwon Sui (year of the dragon)

He died on November 18, 1996 at the age of 92.

AUTHOR'S NOTE

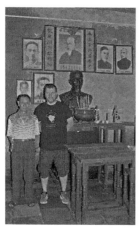
Chan Heung's house

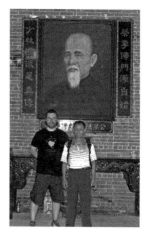
Ancestral school of Chan Heung

Before all I want to thank the fact that he has trusted me and decided to obtain this book, I hope you liked it and fulfilled your expectations.

This book is the first of a very ambitious project based in the publishment of the main forms of the Choy Lee Fut system, with the objective of willing to help the practitioners of this incredible system in their study, for the understanding of the forms along with the acquirement of a vocabulary of indispensable technical terms.

The poetical names of the movements are a fruit of the oral transmission of the forms as well as the hard work of my master Sifu Pun, In order to collect and organize the manuscripts and notes of the teachings transmitted by the GM Chan Yiu Chi.

My contribution in this long way of preserving the system and to transmit it to the next generations is based on my teaching job with my students and instructors, along with the translation and collection of the GM Chan Yiu Chi manuscripts.

This book and those that I hope to publish in the near future have the objective of providing my students and all martial arts practitioners with a bibliography to support during their martial path.

Finally I thank with all my heart their trust and I hope you enjoy the reading and study.

ABOUT AUTHOR

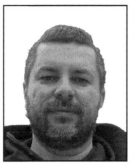

蔡李佛拳第六代传人路易斯先生

Sifu Luis Lázaro 6th generation of the Choy Lee Fut, s the fourth disciple and the only western of Sifu Pun, he dedicates his life for the publishment of the Hung Sing Choy Lee Fut 雄勝蔡李佛 system that was transmitted by the GM Chan Yiu Chi grandson, founder of the Chan Heung.

He started training martial arts at the age of thirteen inside of the Shotokan Karate system, due to his college studies of Senior Chemical Engineering in the Rovira and Virgili of Tarragona University, he stays in the road of the martial arts, this time inside of the Kun-Tao system, system of which he will dedicate more than 6 years.

Once his universities studies finished he starts his studies on traditional chinese medicine and his Choy Lee Fut training, dedicating more than 18 years to it.

In 2014 he becomes a student of Sifu Pun, on which through trainings with closed doors in Guang Zhou he refines and deepens in the Siu Muy Fa Kyun form, and the basis of the Choy Lee Fut system.

In 2015 and 2017 Sifu Pun travels to Tarragona where he stays in the house of Sifu Luis Lázaro and for more than 15 days they execute trainings with doors closed, open seminaries in the Valls, Barcelona and Zaragoza schools; along with trainings with advanced students.

In 2016 on his visit to Guang Zhou, he receives the great gift of being the fourth disciple of Sifu Pun, the day of the celebration of the 210th anniversary of the Chan Heung birthday.

Sifu Luis Lázaro travels every year to China where he spends long stays in order to train in a private way with Sifu Pun.

B

Baai Fat Sik 拜佛式: reverence to the Buddha
Bei Sik 备式: prepared

C

Chaang Geuk 撑脚: kick that crushes
Chaang Jeung 撑掌: palm that crushes
Cheung Ngaam Cheui 抢眼槌: fist to the eye
Chin Si Ma 缠丝马: silk rolling horse
Chuk Yiu 束腰: pick up to the waist

D

Da Geuk 打脚: to kick
Daai Paang 大鹏: great bird
Daap Ma 蹬马:: horse that step
Dai Nau Ma 低扭马: low twist horse
Dei 地: earth
Ding Jeung 顶掌: palm upwards
Ding Ji Ma 丁字马: Ding 丁 character horse
Duk Geuk 独脚: horse of one leg

F

Faan Jong 反撞: hook
Fat Jeung 佛掌: palm of Buddha
Fu 虎: tiger
Fu Jaau 虎爪: tiger claw
Fung Wong 凤凰: golden rooster

G

Gun Yam 观音: buddhist goddess
Gung Kiu 攻桥: bridge that attacks
Gwa Cheui 挂槌: fist that hangs

H

Ha Daan Tin 下丹田: low Daan Tin
Hap Geuk 合脚: feet together
HEI MA 起马: lift the horse
Hoi Ma 开马: open the horse
Hok 鹤: crane
Hok Jeui 鹤咀: crane's peak
Hung Bou 胸部: chest

J
Jaam Jong 站桩: to hug the tree
Jaau 爪: claw
Jeung Sam 掌心: heart of the palm
Jin Cheui 箭槌: arrow fist
Jin Ji 箭指: arrow fingers
Jyu Lung 珠龙: the dragon grabs the pearl

L
Lap Kiu 攬桥: to take the kiu
Luk Kiu 碌桥: to control the rocky bridge
Lung 龙: dragon

K
Kap Cheui 扱槌: fist that stamps a seal

N
Nak Kiu 扐桥: bridge that grabs
Nau Ma 扭马: twisted horse
Ngaat 压: to press

P
Paau 豹: leopard
Pun Kiu 蟠桥: bridge that twists

S
Sang Gung 生弓: the arm as an arc, with fingers pointing to the ear
Sat Ma 实马: real horse
Sau Ma 收马: to lit the horse
Sau Sik 收式: final position
Se 蛇: snake
Sei Ping Ma 四平马: horse of four distances on level
Seung But Kiu 双拔桥: both hands disperse
Seung Chung Jong 双冲撞: raise both elbows by taking the fists to the chest
Seung Gam Jin 上金剪: Golden scissors to the top
Seung Ha Chaang Yut Jeung 双下撑月掌: two palms hold the earth
Seung Jaau 双爪: double claws
Seung Seui Sau 双垂手:: two palms to the sides
Seung Taat Jeung 双挞掌: two palms of whip
Seung Teui Jeung 双推掌: to push with both palms
Siu Lam Ji 少林寺: Shaolin temple

Sou Geuk 扫脚: kick that sweeps

T
Teui Jeung 推掌: push with the palms
Tin 天: sky
Tou Bou 肚部: abdomen

W
Waang Chaang Geuk 橫撐腳: horizontal kick that crushes

Manufactured by Amazon.ca
Bolton, ON